ALISON M HUGHES

Fertility on a Budget

How to Fund IVF, Stay Sane, and Plan Your Path to Parenthood

Copyright © 2025 by Alison M Hughes

All rights reserved. No part of this publication may be reproduced, stored or transmitted in any form or by any means, electronic, mechanical, photocopying, recording, scanning, or otherwise without written permission from the publisher. It is illegal to copy this book, post it to a website, or distribute it by any other means without permission.

Alison M Hughes asserts the moral right to be identified as the author of this work.

Alison M Hughes has no responsibility for the persistence or accuracy of URLs for external or third-party Internet Websites referred to in this publication and does not guarantee that any content on such Websites is, or will remain, accurate or appropriate.

Designations used by companies to distinguish their products are often claimed as trademarks. All brand names and product names used in this book and on its cover are trade names, service marks, trademarks and registered trademarks of their respective owners. The publishers and the book are not associated with any product or vendor mentioned in this book. None of the companies referenced within the book have endorsed the book.

First edition

This book was professionally typeset on Reedsy.
Find out more at reedsy.com

Contents

1	Introduction – Hope Is Not a Luxury	1
2	The IVF Price Tag: Unwrapped	9
3	How People Actually Pay for IVF	24
4	The Fertility Budget Blueprint	39
5	Creative Income Strategies That Don't Burn You Out	50
6	The Power of Boundaries: Saying No Without Guilt	63
7	The Waiting Room: Coping with Delays, Disappointment, and…	77
8	The Informed Patient: How to Advocate for Yourself Without…	89
9	Know Your Rights: Understanding Your Protections, Policies,…	102
10	Staying Connected: Reclaiming Your Body, Identity, and Power…	117
11	Embracing the Path Ahead: Redefining Hope, Family, and…	128
12	The Journey You've Taken, and the One Still to Come	138
13	A Note from the Author	141

1

Introduction - Hope Is Not a Luxury

There's a moment many people facing infertility never forget. It might be the first time they see a fertility specialist's quote printed neatly in a folder. It might be the total cost of one IVF cycle, circled in red: $12,000... $17,000... $23,000. And for some, it's the crushing silence when they realise insurance won't cover any of it.

That moment can feel like the floor giving way beneath your feet. Not because you didn't expect IVF to cost money – you did. But because no one told you it might cost as much as a car or a deposit on a home. No one told you that building a family in this way might require spreadsheets, sacrifice, or sheer financial gymnastics. No one told you how hard it might be to grieve what you thought the journey would look like.

But here's what I want to tell you, right from the beginning:

You are not selfish for wanting a child.

You are not irresponsible for wondering how to afford it.

And you are absolutely not alone.

This book exists for one simple reason: because hope should not be gated by income. Because fertility challenges already carry enormous emotional weight - and we need better support when they carry a financial one, too.

A Silent Struggle with a High Price Tag

Infertility is often a silent, invisible struggle. On the surface, everything looks "normal." You're going to work. You're smiling at friends' baby showers. You're telling yourself to stay optimistic. But beneath that, a whole storm of questions may be raging:

- *Can we really afford this?*
- *How many cycles will we need?*
- *Is it selfish to spend this money?*
- *What if we drain our savings and it still doesn't work?*

These are not just financial questions. They are moral ones. Identity-shaping ones. And they deserve thoughtful, shame-free answers.

Yet most fertility books skip this part. They talk about the medical science, or the emotions, or even the logistics - but they leave the "money talk" for last. If they include it at all, it's a short chapter with vague advice like "check with your insurance provider" or "consider crowdfunding."

That's not good enough.

Because for many people, the financial side is not a footnote. It's the first hurdle. The biggest. The one that makes everything else feel hypothetical.

Why I Wrote This Book

Over the past decade, I've worked with hundreds of women, couples, and solo parents navigating everything from miscarriage to surrogacy, IVF to adoption. And time and again, the same themes emerge: emotional exhaustion, logistical overwhelm, and financial paralysis.

Not because people are bad at managing money. Not because they haven't tried. But because the systems weren't built with them in mind. Because fertility clinics often function more like private businesses than medical partners. Because costs are opaque and uneven. Because some of the most essential decisions - like whether to try one more cycle - come down to whether a credit card can handle it.

So this book is not a lecture on personal finance. It's a bridge. From despair to planning. From sticker shock to strategy. From feeling like this dream is slipping away to realizing: *You may not be able to control the outcome, but you can control the path.*

This book exists because no one should be forced to choose between a baby and bankruptcy. And no one should be shamed for wanting both family and financial stability.

What This Book Will and Won't Do

Let's be clear: this book will not guarantee that you'll have a child through IVF. No ethical book can promise that.

But it will give you the tools to:

- Understand exactly what you're paying for (and why)
- Discover funding sources you may not know exist
- Create a step-by-step plan based on your unique situation
- Build a budget that respects both your fertility dreams and your future financial health
- Navigate difficult emotions around money, fairness, and control

You won't find one-size-fits-all prescriptions. You will find realistic scenarios, case studies, creative options, and yes - spreadsheets, calculators, and templates. Because empowerment doesn't come from wishful thinking. It comes from knowing your numbers *and* your values.

What this book won't do is make assumptions. I don't know if you're partnered or solo, insured or uninsured, working-class or high-earning but debt-laden. I don't know if you've been trying for five years or five months. That's why every chapter is designed to meet you where you are – and offer a menu of possibilities, not a single prescription.

Reclaiming Financial Dignity

There is a myth – unspoken but widespread – that financial worry should come second to fertility. That if you *really* want a baby, you'll "find the money." That talking about budgets or funding options is somehow less romantic, less pure, or less deserving.

Let's dismantle that myth right now.

You can be deeply devoted to having a child and still want to keep your house.

You can love the idea of motherhood and still hate the idea of five-figure debt.

You can be smart, strategic, and emotionally grounded – all at once.

Financial dignity is not about denying your dream. It's about protecting your foundation so that dream can grow.

And the truth is, many people find this process brings out

strengths they didn't know they had. Resourcefulness. Resilience. Creativity. Boundaries. Conversations that once felt taboo - about money, about risk, about compromise - become the scaffolding for the family they go on to build.

What You Can Expect from This Journey

This book is broken into ten chapters, each tackling a key question along your fertility + finance journey:

1. What am I really paying for?
2. How do people actually afford IVF?
3. How can I build a realistic, compassionate budget?
4. Can I earn more (without burning out)?
5. What grants, charities, and "free money" exist?
6. What can my workplace offer (and how do I ask)?
7. Should I travel for more affordable treatment?
8. What happens if a cycle fails - emotionally and financially?
9. How do I plan long-term, no matter the outcome?
10. What does it mean to invest in hope?

Each chapter begins with a story, quote, or real-life scenario to ground the ideas in something human. You'll find tools, tips, and gentle guidance. There will be no guilt-tripping. No unrealistic timelines. And no financial jargon without translation.

There will also be room - room to grieve, to pivot, to celebrate small wins. Because even though this is a book about money, it's also a book about hope. Hope that's planned for. Hope that's protected. Hope that's yours.

One Final Note

I don't know where you are in your journey right now. Maybe you're standing at the very beginning, barely whispering the word IVF out loud. Maybe you're mid-process, reeling from a failed cycle and wondering if you can afford to try again. Maybe you're several cycles in, exhausted by the emotional and financial rollercoaster.

Wherever you are, please know this:

You are not a failure because this is hard.

You are not broken because it's expensive.

You are not alone in wanting to find another way.

This book is yours. To dog-ear, to annotate, to throw across the room and come back to later. I wrote it to help you feel less alone, more prepared, and more powerful. And if nothing else, I hope it reminds you:

You are allowed to want a baby.

You are allowed to talk about money.

You are allowed to do both, with heart and strategy.

Now let's begin.

Alison
 x

2

The IVF Price Tag: Unwrapped

"*Would you pay $20,000 for something you can't guarantee will work?*"

When we talk about IVF costs, the first thing most people think is: *Wait, how can one cycle be that expensive?* And the truth is, most people never see the full breakdown until they're knee-deep in the process. Unlike other major purchases - like a car or a home - IVF doesn't come with a clean itemized receipt upfront. The total cost hides in layers: labs, medications, monitoring, clinic fees, and often unexpected add-ons.

Understanding where your money actually goes is the first and most empowering step in making this process financially manageable. You are not just writing checks - you are making choices. And when those choices are based on real clarity instead of confusion or panic, the emotional burden of IVF becomes just a little lighter.

At its most basic, an IVF cycle includes a predictable sequence of clinical steps. Each step comes with its own fee, and together they form what's often referred to as the "base cost." Depending on your location and clinic, this can range from $10,000 to $20,000 before medication or optional extras.

It starts with initial consultations and diagnostics. These usually include a fertility assessment for both partners (or just one, in the case of solo parenting), hormonal bloodwork to assess ovarian reserve and cycle timing, ultrasounds to evaluate the uterus and ovaries, and semen analysis if needed. Some clinics also recommend genetic carrier screening, especially if there's a family history of inherited conditions. These steps aren't just formalities - they shape the entire treatment plan. But even at this early stage, the costs start to build.

Next comes ovarian stimulation and monitoring. You'll be prescribed a specific protocol - a tailored combination of hormonal injections to encourage your ovaries to produce multiple eggs. While you're doing this at home each day, you'll be returning to the clinic frequently - often every second day - for blood tests and internal ultrasounds to monitor how your body is responding. Adjustments are often made along the way to balance effectiveness and safety. These monitoring visits are essential, but they're often priced separately from the base cycle fee.

Then comes the egg retrieval. This is a minor surgical procedure done under sedation, often in the clinic's surgical suite. It's quick - typically under an hour - but it involves specialized equipment, an anesthesiologist, and a lab team ready to process your eggs on the spot. Once retrieved, the eggs are passed along to the embryologist, who fertilizes them in the lab with sperm - either from a partner or a donor. Embryo development over the next five days is carefully tracked, often with optional time-lapse imaging systems that some clinics recommend for an extra cost. The quality of embryos is assessed and graded.

If all goes well, you'll return for an embryo transfer. This involves placing a selected embryo into the uterus using ultrasound guidance. The procedure is generally quick and painless, but again, it carries separate clinical fees, along with follow-up testing to confirm whether implantation was successful.

Along the way, you may also encounter administrative fees - coordination charges, medication handling, medical records requests, or separate billing for anesthesia. While each fee may seem minor in isolation, they can accumulate quickly, and they're rarely advertised upfront.

But the biggest wildcard in your IVF bill? Medications.

Medication costs are rarely included in the "cycle price" quoted by clinics, and yet they can run between $3,000 and $7,000 per cycle - sometimes more. The drugs you'll need depend on your protocol, and some people require higher doses than others due to age, ovarian reserve, or previous response.

These aren't medications you can pick up at your local pharmacy. They're often specialty injectables requiring refrigeration, time-sensitive shipping, and precise administration. Brand-name drugs dominate the market, and generics - when available - can still be pricey. Insurance coverage is inconsistent at best. Many policies that cover the procedure do not cover the medications.

You might use drugs like Gonal-F or Menopur to stimulate

egg production, Lupron or Cetrotide to suppress premature ovulation, and then Ovidrel to trigger final maturation before retrieval. After transfer, progesterone support - often in the form of injections or suppositories - is essential to help maintain the uterine lining. Each of these medications has a cost. Often, that cost fluctuates depending on your location, your chosen pharmacy, and how much price comparison you're willing - or able - to do while managing the emotional weight of treatment.

There are ways to reduce medication costs. Compounding pharmacies may offer lower prices on certain injectables. Some clinics work with pharmaceutical discount programs or shared medication programs. International pharmacies are sometimes cheaper, but shipping timelines can be unpredictable. One woman I spoke to called seven different pharmacies across three states, ultimately saving $2,000 on her protocol by finding a lesser-known local supplier who agreed to match a discount card price.

Beyond the essentials, you'll be presented with optional add-ons. This is where costs can increase dramatically - and where it becomes especially important to distinguish between medical necessity and clinic preference.

Preimplantation genetic testing is a common example. PGT-A screens embryos for chromosomal abnormalities, potentially lowering miscarriage risk or helping identify which embryos to transfer first. PGT-M, a separate test, checks for single-gene disorders if you or your partner carry a known condition. These tests can add between $3,000 and $7,000 to your bill, depending on the number of embryos and which lab is used. While these technologies can offer peace of mind - and sometimes improve outcomes - they are not universally necessary. For younger patients with no known genetic risks, the cost may outweigh the benefit. But clinics don't always make that distinction clear.

Embryo freezing is another cost to consider. If you have surplus embryos, you may want to preserve them for future cycles. Freezing can add $1,000 to $2,000 to the cycle, with annual storage fees of $350 to $1,000. Some clinics outsource storage, while others handle it in-house. It's a valuable option - it can save you the emotional and physical toll of a second full cycle - but it's not always bundled into the quoted package.

And then there are wellness extras. "Embryo glue" to aid implantation. Acupuncture packages. Proprietary supplements. Special uterine receptivity testing. Time-lapse embryo imaging systems with high-tech cameras. These add-ons are often framed as small advantages - a few hundred dollars here, another test there - but they can quickly add thousands to your total cost, often with limited or conflicting evidence of improved outcomes.

A single woman I worked with made the decision to skip genetic testing and instead split her savings across two smaller cycles - what some clinics call "mini IVF." With a little luck and good timing, she ended up with two healthy embryos and a successful transfer on her second try. What she gained was not just savings, but peace of mind that her budget was being used where it mattered most to her.

This is not about rejecting science or saying no to helpful interventions. It's about making sure every dollar you spend reflects your values, your medical reality, and your financial boundaries.

Because once you see the full picture, something powerful happens: the fear starts to shrink. You begin to ask better questions. You start to realize that this isn't just something happening to you – it's something you're actively shaping.

You don't need to memorize every medical term or become an accountant. You just need to know enough to advocate for yourself. And to recognize that "more expensive" doesn't always mean "more effective."

Just because a clinic charges more doesn't mean it offers better results. And just because you're budgeting doesn't mean you're settling. In the next chapter, we'll look at how to compare clinics without losing your mind – or your financial footing.

Because understanding the price is one thing. Understanding the value? That's where real power begins.

Choosing Wisely: Comparing Clinics Without Losing Your Mind

When you're facing down the cost of IVF, one of the first major decisions you'll make is where to undergo treatment. And it's not a simple choice. Fertility clinics are not all created equal – not in price, not in approach, and certainly not in transparency. Some people feel lucky if there's even one clinic nearby; others are overwhelmed with choices in major metro areas. Either way, choosing a clinic isn't just a medical decision. It's a financial, emotional, and logistical one too.

What makes this particularly challenging is that many clinics present their services like retail packages: tiered pricing, flashy success rates, bundled offers, and add-on "upgrades" that blur the lines between medical care and marketing. And that can be exhausting when all you're trying to do is build a family without losing your financial footing.

So how do you compare clinics wisely - without losing your clarity, your courage, or your budget? The answer begins with looking beneath the surface.

The first thing to understand is the difference between *cost-per-cycle* and *cost-per-live-birth.* Many clinics advertise a competitive price for one cycle, but that number is only a fraction of the real cost if that first cycle doesn't lead to a pregnancy. National averages show that many people need more than one cycle to conceive - and when you factor in medication, add-ons, and recovery time, that number can climb quickly.

That's why the smarter question to ask is: *What will this clinic actually cost me to have a baby, not just to try for one?* Some clinics with slightly higher upfront costs may actually offer better value - not because they promise better odds, but because they provide more comprehensive care, more transparent pricing, or higher cumulative success rates.

It helps to look beyond the marketing language. Most clinics highlight their "success rates," but these numbers can be presented in misleading ways. For example, some clinics report only clinical pregnancies (a positive test), not live births. Others may exclude older patients or higher-risk cases from their published stats to keep their numbers impressive.

To compare fairly, go directly to the source: the CDC and SART (Society for Assisted Reproductive Technology) both publish public data on IVF clinics in the U.S. These databases include live birth rates by age group, type of treatment, and even number of embryos transferred. It takes time to sift through, but it's well worth it. You're not just looking for the flashiest number – you're looking for consistent, honest reporting and solid outcomes for people like you.

Then there's location. It's tempting to go with the closest clinic – and sometimes that really is the best choice. But depending on your flexibility, you may find that traveling even a few hours away opens the door to better options. In many parts of the country, urban centers are saturated with high-priced clinics, while smaller regional centers offer similar success rates for thousands less per cycle. That's not always true – but it's worth exploring. The key is balancing what's practical with what's possible.

One couple I interviewed lived in a mid-sized town with one well-known clinic charging $22,000 per cycle. After some digging, they discovered a smaller clinic in a neighboring state with excellent success rates and a price tag closer to $14,000. Factoring in travel costs and time off work, they still saved nearly $6,000 – and felt better supported during the process because of the clinic's smaller, more personal environment.

Of course, money isn't the only metric that matters. How a clinic makes you feel matters, too. IVF is intimate. Vulnerable. Personal. You deserve to be treated like a human being – not a number or a transaction. If the front desk staff seem rushed, if communication is unclear, or if your questions are brushed aside during your initial consult, that's not something to dismiss. That's data.

During your first consultation - whether in person or virtual - pay attention to more than just the price sheet. Ask yourself:

- Are they explaining the process in a way that makes sense?
- Do they offer cost transparency upfront?
- Are they pushing expensive add-ons too early?
- Do they welcome your questions?
- Do you feel heard?

These "soft signals" are not trivial. In fact, they're often the best indicators of whether you'll feel supported throughout a long, emotionally complex process. A clinic that truly respects your financial boundaries will be clear about what's required, what's optional, and what might work for *you*, not just for their averages.

Don't be afraid to get multiple consultations. In other areas of healthcare, we routinely get second opinions - and you're allowed to do that here too. In fact, some clinics offer free or discounted initial consults, especially if you ask. Think of it as dating before marriage. You wouldn't commit thousands of dollars and months of your life to someone after one meeting - the same standard should apply to your clinic.

Another important point: ask for an itemized quote. Many clinics will give you a packaged number that sounds convenient

- "$17,500 for a complete cycle!" - but the details might reveal that medications, monitoring, or lab work aren't included. Others may offer "all-inclusive" packages that sound generous, but quietly exclude certain common procedures, like ICSI or embryo freezing.

An itemized breakdown gives you negotiating power. It also allows you to compare apples to apples when looking at different clinics. You'll quickly notice that one clinic might charge $6,000 for lab fees while another charges $2,500. That kind of discrepancy matters.

Be mindful, too, of refund or shared-risk programs. Some clinics offer a "money-back guarantee" if IVF doesn't work after a set number of cycles - but these usually come at a much higher upfront cost. These programs can offer peace of mind, especially for people who qualify easily, but they can also be financially risky if you don't meet the refund criteria (which are often stricter than advertised). Read the fine print, and be wary of emotionally persuasive language like "guaranteed baby" or "no-risk success."

You deserve a clinic that treats you with dignity, transparency, and care. That doesn't always mean choosing the most expensive option or the one with the flashiest building. It means choosing a place where your emotional, physical, and financial wellbeing are all respected.

This part of the process - the choosing - is not a detour. It's part of the journey. When you make a choice that aligns with your values and resources, you begin your IVF process not from a place of desperation, but from a place of quiet power.

Because clarity is strength. And being a patient doesn't mean giving up your role as a decision-maker.

Next, we'll take a closer look at what role insurance really plays in all this - and how to find out what's actually covered versus what's quietly excluded. Because the fine print? It matters more than most people realise.

Reading the Fine Print: What Insurance Really Covers

One of the most common - and most emotionally charged - questions people ask at the start of their fertility journey is: *Does my insurance cover any of this?* It's a question asked with hope, with dread, and with genuine confusion. Because in many cases, the answer isn't a simple yes or no - it's a hesitant, deeply buried *"sort of."*

The reality is that fertility coverage is a patchwork: uneven, inconsistent, and often filled with frustrating loopholes. Some people are lucky enough to have generous plans that cover multiple cycles, medication, and monitoring. Others find out, usually too late, that they're responsible for every penny - even though their plan technically claims to offer "fertility benefits."

Let's pull back the curtain on this complicated landscape. Because understanding what your insurance *actually* covers can help you avoid unexpected costs, challenge unfair denials, and plan smarter from the beginning.

Many insurance policies - especially in the U.S. - use broad, vague language when it comes to fertility care. You might read phrases like "diagnostic testing covered" or "infertility services eligible under certain conditions." But what does that mean in practice?

For many plans, there's a crucial distinction between *diagnosis* and *treatment*. In other words, your insurance might pay for the process of *finding out* why you're not conceiving - blood tests, ultrasounds, even a semen analysis - but not for the actual treatment that follows, such as IVF or IUI. This creates a deeply frustrating dynamic: you're allowed to know what's wrong, but you're on your own to fix it.

To add to the confusion, some plans include language requiring a "failure to conceive naturally" for a certain period of time - often one year for heterosexual couples, or six months if the birthing partner is over 35. For LGBTQ+ couples or single parents by choice, this can lead to outright denial unless they undergo (and pay for) multiple rounds of insemination to prove "infertility," even when biology makes natural conception impossible.

This is not just a bureaucratic glitch. It's a form of exclusion - and it can be profoundly disheartening.
But there are ways to push back.

The first step is to get your full plan details in writing. Not just the summary - the full policy. You can request this from your HR department or your insurer directly. Once you have it, look for the specific terms under sections like "infertility services," "reproductive health," or "excluded procedures."
Be prepared for language that's dry and technical. That's okay.

Highlight any phrases you don't understand and bring them to a benefits coordinator or patient advocate - either through your clinic or through an independent fertility support group.

Don't be afraid to ask the hard questions:

- Does this plan cover IVF? If so, how many cycles?
- Are medications included?
- Is prior authorization required, and if so, what does that involve?
- Are there prerequisites (such as documented infertility or age limits)?
- Does it cover procedures for same-sex couples or single parents?

Sometimes, plans appear to exclude IVF but do cover parts of the process - like diagnostic testing, lab work, or even medications. These partial coverages can still offer meaningful savings if you know how to access them.

In some cases, appealing a denial is possible - and successful. If your doctor can demonstrate that IVF is medically necessary, you may be able to obtain an exception. Supporting letters from your physician, combined with a written personal statement, can be powerful. Clinics often have staff who help with appeals - ask them early and often.

It's also worth knowing that a growing number of states in the U.S. have mandates requiring insurers to offer some level of fertility coverage. As of now, around 20 states have laws on the books - but the specifics vary widely. Some require only diagnostic testing; others require full coverage of IVF under certain conditions. A handful include egg freezing for medical reasons. Most states, however, still don't require insurers to cover fertility at all.

If you live in a mandated state, know your rights. Employers and insurers don't always volunteer this information, so being informed is your best defense. You can find up-to-date state-by-state guides through RESOLVE: The National Infertility Association.

Beyond the insurance card in your wallet, it's also worth looking at other pathways to coverage. Some employers offer fertility benefits not through traditional insurance, but through third-party fertility programs like Progyny, Carrot, or WINFertility. These platforms often provide bundled services - including treatment navigation, medication discounts, and emotional support - as part of your workplace perks, even if standard insurance doesn't.

Ask your HR department directly: *Do we have any partnerships with fertility benefit providers?* These programs are increasingly common in large companies, tech firms, healthcare systems, and financial organizations. They're also becoming a quiet recruitment tool - a fact worth leveraging, especially if you're considering changing jobs to support your family-building goals.

One woman I spoke with worked for a retail company that didn't appear to offer any fertility benefits. But after she reached out to HR, she discovered the company had recently added a third-party fertility benefit - and just hadn't announced it yet. She ended up accessing two full IVF cycles through the program, saving nearly $40,000 in the process.

Stories like that remind us that clarity doesn't just save money - it can open doors we didn't even know existed.

If your insurance offers no meaningful coverage - or if you're uninsured altogether - it's not the end of the road. Many people build families without coverage, using a mix of grants, budgeting strategies, employer perks, and creative planning. And you'll find every one of those options in the chapters ahead.

Still, there's something deeply validating about knowing your plan. Even if the answer is disappointing, even if coverage is denied, you've moved from vague fear into informed action.

You deserve to know what's on the table. And you deserve care that sees your whole story - not just your lab results.

In the next chapter, we'll explore how people actually pay for IVF - the practical, emotional, and creative funding paths that make treatment possible, even when insurance isn't part of the picture.

3

How People Actually Pay for IVF

"*It's not all savings and second mortgages – some of the best resources are hiding in plain sight.*"

When the doctor tells you the cost of one IVF cycle – and then gently reminds you it often takes more than one – there's usually a long pause. A quiet, stunned kind of silence. Most people don't respond right away. Not because they don't care, but because they're calculating. Silently, inwardly, anxiously. *How...?*

There's this strange cultural belief that people who do IVF are somehow wealthy – or at the very least, unusually financially stable. But that's not true. Most people pursuing fertility treatment are regular people trying to build a family, not buy a luxury car. They have bills, rent, mortgages, student loans, childcare costs, and aging parents. And they're often doing all of this while carrying the invisible emotional weight of loss, uncertainty, and decision fatigue.

So how do people actually pay for IVF?

The short answer: every way you can imagine. And the long answer? That's what this chapter is about.

There is no single path. Some people save methodically for years. Others piece together funding from five or six different sources. Many use a mix of traditional strategies and creative workarounds, and just as many learn by doing – one invoice, one medication bill, one difficult choice at a time.

Let's walk through what those funding paths look like. Not just the ones we assume are out there, but the ones you might not yet know exist.

Most people begin with the usual suspects. They dip into savings, if they have any. They might take out a personal loan, apply for a medical financing plan, or reach for a credit card – even if the interest makes their stomach turn. Some lean on family. Some sell assets, take on extra work, or rearrange their budgets. And some do all of the above, cobbling together their dream with more determination than anyone gives them credit for.

There's nothing wrong with these options. In fact, when handled with awareness and support, they can be lifesaving. But they're not the only way – and for many, they're not sustainable long-term. High-interest debt can turn an already emotional process into a pressure cooker. And saving $20,000 in a hurry? That's not a reasonable ask for most families.

That's why it's essential to look beyond the obvious. There are overlooked lifelines that many people never explore – not because they don't qualify, but because they simply didn't know where to look.

One of the most underutilized resources is your employer.

More companies than ever now offer fertility benefits - even if they don't advertise them. These aren't always obvious. They might be tucked into your health plan, offered through a separate fertility partner (like Progyny or WINFertility), or available as part of a wellness or flexible spending package. Some employers also offer adoption or surrogacy stipends that can, with the right documentation, be used toward IVF or embryo preservation.

If your employer doesn't currently offer fertility benefits, that doesn't mean it's a dead end. Some employees have successfully advocated for benefits to be added, especially if they're in companies that prioritize inclusion and family-friendly policies. Your voice matters more than you think - especially when combined with others. Quietly asking HR what might be available is not only reasonable, it's strategic.

Another overlooked lifeline? Health Savings Accounts (HSAs) and Flexible Spending Accounts (FSAs). If you have one of these accounts through your employer or a private plan, you may be able to use pre-tax dollars to pay for many aspects of fertility treatment - including medication, diagnostic testing, and some procedures. That can mean instant savings of 20–30%, depending on your tax bracket.

Then there are discount programs, grants, and patient-assistance offerings from pharmaceutical companies. Many fertility medication manufacturers have income-based programs that reduce or even eliminate medication costs. Clinics themselves sometimes have sliding-scale programs, or offer discounts to military families, cancer survivors, LGBTQ+ patients, or teachers and nurses. These aren't always publicized

– you have to ask.

There's also medical tourism – choosing to travel for treatment, either within your own country or abroad. Some families save thousands by receiving care in reputable international clinics where quality is high and cost is lower. We'll explore this option in more depth later in the book, but for now it's worth holding the idea with curiosity, not fear.

And then, of course, there's crowdfunding. This one carries mixed feelings for many – pride, vulnerability, even guilt. But let's reframe it: asking for help isn't weakness. It's honesty. IVF is a medical treatment. If someone you loved were diagnosed with cancer and needed help paying for surgery, would you judge them for creating a GoFundMe? Probably not. You'd say they're brave.

People want to help you. And when you share your story authentically – with dignity, without pressure – you give others the opportunity to show up for you. Some couples have funded their entire treatment through crowdfunding; others simply raised enough for one medication refill or one ultrasound. That counts too.

One woman I know launched a small Etsy store selling handmade fertility affirmation cards. She started it as a side project during her first cycle, hoping to raise a few hundred dollars. Over time, it turned into a business – and she used the profits to pay for her second round of IVF. She told me later, "It helped me feel like I was part of my own solution, not just waiting and worrying."

That's the real heart of this chapter: you are allowed to get creative. You are allowed to build your family *your* way, using every resource you can find. There is no single "respectable" way to pay for IVF. There is only what works for you, your body, your values, and your bank account.

You may need to mix and match. You may need to pause and re-strategize. And yes - you may have to have uncomfortable conversations with people you love. But every single family built through IVF was once just a person sitting in a clinic, staring at the cost, and wondering how to make it work.

You are not behind. You are not doing it wrong. You are doing something brave and resourceful and emotionally complex - and you are allowed to find a way forward that doesn't wreck your financial future in the process.

In the next chapter, we'll turn all of this information into something tangible. We'll build a realistic, compassionate, and flexible fertility budget - one that makes space not just for bills and medication, but for the life you want to live while pursuing the family you're dreaming of.

The Overlooked Lifelines

When people think of paying for IVF, their minds often jump to big-ticket strategies - dipping into savings, taking out loans, maxing credit cards, or remortgaging their home. But behind the scenes, many hopeful parents are funding their treatment with a much more intricate patchwork of resources. Quietly. Creatively. Often invisibly.

These overlooked lifelines don't always show up in the glossy brochures or clinic websites. They may not feel "official," and they almost never come with neon signs saying *This will save you thousands!* But they're real – and for many people, they've been the bridge between "we can't afford this" and "we're giving it a shot."

One of the most underutilized resources? Your own workplace.

Many employees never think to ask whether their employer offers fertility benefits. They assume that if it's not loudly advertised, it must not exist. But fertility coverage is often buried in HR manuals, health plan riders, or third-party vendor partnerships – and it's not always presented as "IVF coverage." It might be called "family-building support," "wellness reimbursement," or even "reproductive services."

Some companies now work with organizations like **Carrot**, **WIN-Fertility**, or **Progyny**, which handle everything from treatment navigation to medication discounts. These partnerships are separate from your main health insurance and can exist quietly in the background until you ask.

One woman I spoke with worked in HR for a healthcare system that didn't publicize any fertility benefits. But after she pressed for clarity, she discovered her employer had recently added a Progyny plan with generous IVF coverage. It simply hadn't been announced yet. She went from assuming she'd have to pay $25,000 out of pocket to discovering she qualified for multiple cycles under her employee plan – a game-changer.

Even if your workplace doesn't offer formal coverage, some companies will reimburse parts of the process through **flexible**

benefits. That might include reimbursing travel to a clinic, supporting time off during procedures, or covering certain medications through a **health reimbursement arrangement (HRA)**. Every policy is different, but every question asked opens a door.

Then there's the power of **tax-advantaged spending accounts** - like **HSAs (Health Savings Accounts)** and **FSAs (Flexible Spending Accounts)**. If you have one of these through your employer or a private insurance plan, don't overlook it. These accounts allow you to use **pre-tax dollars** to pay for qualified medical expenses, which may include fertility testing, monitoring, medication, and sometimes even parts of the procedure itself. That's an immediate savings of 20–30% depending on your tax bracket.

Many people underestimate how much they can use these accounts for. Yes, the rules vary depending on the provider and the type of treatment, but even if IVF itself isn't covered, the surrounding services might be. That includes:

- Diagnostic testing
- Hormone therapy
- Embryology lab work
- Blood draws
- Ultrasounds
- Fertility-related medications

A simple call to your HSA/FSA administrator, or a visit to your patient portal, can clarify what's eligible and how to get reimbursed.

Medication savings are another lifeline people often miss - not because they don't care, but because it's hard to comparison shop when you're grieving or overwhelmed. Fertility medications can cost anywhere from $3,000 to $7,000 per cycle, but not all pharmacies charge the same price. Specialty pharmacies, online suppliers, and **international vendors** may offer substantial savings - sometimes hundreds or even thousands of dollars less for the exact same drugs.

It's also worth knowing that **pharmaceutical companies themselves** often offer income-based discount programs. These are designed to support patients who are uninsured, underinsured, or struggling with costs - and they're not always widely promoted. The forms can be a little daunting, but clinics often have coordinators who can help you complete them.

Some examples include:

- **Compassionate Care Program** (EMD Serono): Discounts on Gonal-F and other injectables based on income
- **Ferring's Heart Beat Program**: Fertility meds for cancer patients undergoing preservation
- **First Steps Program** (DesignRx): Sliding-scale discounts for select medications

Even if you think you won't qualify, it's worth applying. Discounts range from 10% to 75%, and in rare cases, patients receive medications free of charge.

There's also the option of **shared medication programs**, where leftover unopened medications are donated or sold at a discount through fertility support groups or patient communities. While this is a more informal path - and one that comes with caveats around safety and legality - it's another example of how community can step in when the system fails to provide.

In some areas, local nonprofits and community foundations offer microgrants for fertility care - especially for teachers, veterans, LGBTQ+ families, and people facing cancer or other medical conditions. These grants may not cover the whole cycle, but they can ease the pressure of a medication bill or help offset travel costs. You won't always find them through a basic internet search, so consider connecting with national organizations like RESOLVE or the Tinina Q. Cade Foundation, who often maintain updated grant lists.

Some clinics themselves quietly offer **internal financial assistance** or reduced pricing based on income, medical need, or special circumstances - but they don't always advertise it. You may need to ask directly, respectfully, and persistently. A patient advocate, financial counselor, or even your doctor may be able to authorize lower-cost options - especially if you've built a trusting relationship with the care team.

One couple I interviewed had been saving for a year and were still $5,000 short of the cost of treatment. When they spoke with their clinic's billing coordinator and explained their situation, the clinic offered them a flexible payment plan with no interest - something that wasn't listed anywhere on the website. "They saw we were serious," the woman said. "And they met us halfway. We never would've known if we hadn't asked."

That last part is key.

You don't get what you don't ask for.

Sometimes, all it takes is a question. A phone call. A message to HR. A request for an itemized bill. A bit of boldness in the face of systems that can feel rigid or unfair.

You are not greedy for asking. You are not burdensome for needing help. You are navigating one of the most emotionally, physically, and financially demanding medical journeys anyone can take - and you're doing it with thoughtfulness, courage, and care.

Let the system surprise you - in the good way, for once. Ask the question. Press the issue. Advocate for yourself with the same strength you're already using to build your family.

In the next section, we'll explore even more creative - and sometimes unconventional - ways people are covering the cost of IVF, from crowdfunding to side hustles, and even by turning their grief into entrepreneurial gold.

Alternative Paths: Crowdfunding, Community, and Creative Financing

Not every fertility journey fits inside a neat financial box. Even with insurance sleuthing, employer benefits, HSA accounts, and pharmaceutical discounts, there are still many hopeful parents left staring down a gap - between what they have and what IVF costs. That space in between? That's where creativity, courage, and community can quietly change everything.

Let's begin with a method that often carries complicated emotions: **crowdfunding**.

It's no longer unusual to see GoFundMe campaigns in your social media feed. People crowdfund for surgeries, adoptions, even funeral expenses. So why not fertility treatment? IVF is a medical procedure - one that, for many, is every bit as urgent and necessary as any other. And yet, there's still a lingering sense of guilt or embarrassment around asking for help to grow a family.

But here's the truth: asking for help is not weakness. It's vulnerability. And it takes real strength.

Crowdfunding works best when it's personal and authentic. The most successful campaigns are those that tell a clear, heartfelt story - one that invites others into your journey, not just your expenses. You don't need to overshare, and you don't need to justify your pain. But being open about what you're facing, why IVF is part of your path, and what support would mean to you can make a real difference.

Some couples raise thousands. Others raise just enough to cover one medication refill, or the cost of a trigger shot, or travel to and from appointments. That matters too. Every dollar is not just financial - it's emotional. It says: *We see you. We're with you.*

It also helps to pair crowdfunding with **a specific milestone** or expense. For example: "We are trying to raise $3,200 for the medication needed for our first IVF cycle in September." This gives your supporters a tangible sense of what their help will do. Some people offer small thank-you gifts or updates, but it's not essential. Most people give because they care, not because they want something in return.

Outside of crowdfunding platforms, **community-based support** can be surprisingly powerful. Local churches, synagogues, mosques, and other religious communities often have quiet funds for medical hardship, especially when approached with honesty and clarity. These gifts may not be advertised, but they're given - often by people who understand the ache of longing and the desire to build a family.

In addition to religious or cultural institutions, there are growing networks of **fertility support groups**, both online and in-person, that serve not just as emotional havens but as sources of material support. Some groups coordinate medication sharing (within legal limits), organize donation drives, or host local fundraisers. A handful of community-based nonprofits now focus exclusively on fertility access, offering small grants, medication donations, or even transportation stipends to low-income patients.

One woman I spoke with was a member of a small infertility book club in her city. After sharing her financial struggles during a particularly tough cycle, her group quietly banded together to cover the cost of her progesterone supplements - about $600 total. "It wasn't the money that overwhelmed me," she said later. "It was that I didn't have to be strong and silent anymore."

Then there are **shared-risk programs**, offered by some clinics or third-party financing companies. These packages allow you to pay a higher upfront cost in exchange for multiple cycles, or a partial refund if treatment doesn't result in a live birth. On the surface, these offers can sound like a financial safety net - and for some, they are. But they're also not for everyone.

Shared-risk programs typically come with strict eligibility criteria: you may need to be under a certain age, have a specific BMI, meet hormonal thresholds, or be a "good responder" to medications. The terms may exclude certain conditions or limit you to specific labs or timelines. It's important to read the fine print carefully - and to consider whether locking in a high upfront cost is worth the potential payoff.

That said, for those who do qualify, shared-risk programs can ease the emotional and financial burden of "what if it doesn't work?" They can provide psychological breathing room, especially for people who fear having to choose between a second attempt and their mortgage.

Some families also explore **creative financing options**, including IVF-specific personal loans, zero-interest payment plans, and fertility-focused credit programs. These financing tools are sometimes offered directly through clinics, or through platforms like Ally, CapexMD, or Future Family. Each has its own terms, interest rates, and credit requirements, but they all aim to make treatment feel more accessible - even if you don't have cash in hand.

A word of caution: not all financing is created equal. Some loans come with high origination fees, balloon payments, or interest rates that escalate after a promotional period. Before committing to any loan, ask the following:

- What is the total repayment amount (not just the monthly payment)?
- Is there a prepayment penalty?
- Are there fees built into the loan?
- What happens if my cycle is canceled or postponed?

It's easy to say yes when you're emotional. But financial clarity is a form of self-protection - and future-you deserves to be supported just as much as present-you does.

And then there's a whole other category of funding: **creative income**. Whether it's launching a side hustle, selling handmade goods, picking up extra freelance work, or renting out a spare room on Airbnb - some people have found that the answer isn't just in saving better, but in earning smarter.

We'll explore these strategies more deeply in the next chapter. But for now, know this: there is no shame in using the tools you have. Whether that's your story, your skills, your community, or your creativity.

You are allowed to take an unconventional path. You are allowed to be both soft and strategic. And you are allowed to believe that your dream is worth investing in - even if that investment looks different than you once imagined.

In the next chapter, we'll build your **fertility budget blueprint** - a plan that balances emotional readiness with financial realism. You'll learn how to track your costs, plan for flexibility, and design a budget that supports not just your treatment, but your life.

Because this isn't just about affording IVF. It's about *living* while you do.

4

The Fertility Budget Blueprint

"If IVF were a road trip, would you drive blind without checking your fuel or your map?"

There's a moment in nearly every fertility journey when someone opens a spreadsheet, or a clinic invoice, or a slightly crumpled notebook, and quietly mutters, *We need a plan.* Not a vague plan. A real one. With numbers and boundaries and enough breathing room to feel like you can still live your life while you try to grow your family.

That's what this chapter is for. Not to make you a finance expert. Not to guilt you into saving more. But to give you something gentle to hold on to - a clear, flexible, compassionate guide through the money side of IVF.

And we begin with the most important, often-overlooked step: **knowing where you're starting from**.

Budgeting for IVF can feel like trying to pack for a trip you've never taken, with no clear map and a weather forecast that keeps changing. But before you worry about how much to save or where the money will come from, the most grounding thing you can do is take stock of what's already there.

Start by looking gently and honestly at what's coming in and what's going out. That means your monthly income – not just salaries, but side gigs, support payments, passive income, or anything else contributing to your household. Write it all down. There's no number too small to matter. Then look at your expenses. The fixed ones like rent and loan payments. The flexible ones like groceries and childcare. The automatic ones that renew quietly – subscriptions, memberships, services you may have forgotten.

This isn't about cutting. It's about **clarity**. You're not punishing yourself with numbers – you're simply turning anxiety into information. When you subtract what you spend from what you earn, you get a picture of your monthly margin – the money available to set aside or redirect toward your treatment goals. That number, whatever it is, becomes the foundation of your fertility budget.

And if that number is smaller than you'd like? That doesn't make you irresponsible or behind. It just means your plan will need a little more creativity or support. Knowing the number is empowering, even if it's uncomfortable at first.

Once you know your current financial rhythm, the next question is timing. **When** do you hope to begin IVF? And how flexible is that timeline?

Some people have years to plan and save. Others are racing against the clock – whether it's age, a medical diagnosis, or something more intuitive, like the feeling that this chapter in their life needs to start now. Whatever your timeline is, try to define it. Even an estimate – three months, six months, next year – gives you a framework for what's possible.

From there, you can begin to translate your timeline into monthly savings goals. Let's say you estimate needing £12,000 in six months. That's £2,000 per month – a tall order, yes, but one that might become more manageable with grants, flexible payment plans, or medication discounts. If that number feels out of reach, it's not a sign that you're failing. It's a cue to **restructure the plan**, not abandon the dream.

This is where a realistic, flexible fertility budget starts to emerge – one that reflects not only the hard numbers, but the emotional shape of your life.

Because budgeting for IVF isn't just about figuring out how much things cost. It's also about **how you want to feel** as you move through this process. That includes factoring in the cost of recovery days, therapy sessions, extra groceries when cooking feels too hard, or petrol for those countless early-morning clinic appointments.

It also means looking ahead and asking: will you or your partner need time off work? Is it paid? Do you have flexibility, or will you need to save more to cover that lost income? Will you need childcare while you're at appointments or recovering from egg retrieval? These aren't just logistical details. They're emotional ones, too. Planning for them can bring peace of mind when everything else feels up in the air.

And finally, remember that budgeting for IVF is not just a spreadsheet activity. It's **emotional work**. It's looking at your hopes and fears, and translating them into a plan. If you're budgeting with a partner, try to set a regular time each week or month to check in - not just about money, but about how you're both feeling in the process. Some couples light a candle. Others go out for coffee. What matters is the rhythm - the shared space to say: *This is hard. But we're in it together.*

Even if you're going through this alone, that same rhythm applies. Create moments to check in with yourself. Celebrate the small wins - an extra £50 saved, a new funding option discovered, a helpful call with your clinic. Every step counts.

The clarity you're building now will serve you throughout the journey. It doesn't guarantee an outcome - nothing in IVF does. But it **protects your nervous system**. It gives your decisions a scaffold. And it offers a small but mighty sense of control in a process that so often feels out of your hands.

In the next section, we'll look at how to transform these numbers into a working budget - one that aligns with your actual treatment plan, holds space for both flexibility and emotion, and respects your life beyond fertility.

Now that you've gathered the numbers - income, expenses, timeline, and likely costs - it's time to start shaping those into something more tangible. A fertility budget is not just about tracking where money goes. It's a way to put intention behind every choice. It's a plan that says: *I'm not powerless here.*

And unlike many traditional budgets, a fertility budget has to do more than cover costs. It has to carry **grief, hope, uncertainty, and flexibility**. It has to hold both your plan and your pivot.

One of the most effective tools for doing this is a **dedicated fertility fund**. This is a separate account, wallet, or sub-savings goal designed specifically for anything IVF-related – consultations, medication, transport, emotional support, frozen embryo storage. Keeping these funds separate from your day-to-day money reduces confusion, and more importantly, it protects your sense of purpose. You're not just saving. You're investing in a future you're actively working toward.

You don't need a huge deposit to start. In fact, starting small – even symbolically – is powerful. Transfer £25 or £50 into your fund and name it something meaningful. "Baby Savings" or "Hope Fund." Some people use the month they plan to begin treatment. Others use the name of a song, a place, or a future dream. Language matters. It helps you stay emotionally connected when the process feels transactional.

Once your fund is set up, begin sketching out your expected expenses. Start with what you know or can estimate:

- The base cost of one IVF cycle at your chosen clinic
- Medication (which is often billed separately)
- Any extra procedures (like ICSI, embryo freezing, or PGT testing)
- Monitoring appointments and bloodwork
- Travel or accommodation, if you're going out of town
- Counselling, acupuncture, massage, or other support services
- Contingency costs (cycle cancellation, protocol changes, etc.)

Even if some numbers are rough, listing them helps bring shape to the unknown. If your clinic hasn't yet provided a cost breakdown, ask for one. Many have itemised estimates ready, and if not, request a detailed conversation with their billing coordinator. You're not being difficult - you're being prepared.

With your estimates in hand, create a working document. This could be a spreadsheet, a notebook table, or a budgeting app. Include columns for: item, estimated cost, amount saved, and remaining balance. This gives you a living overview - not just of what you owe, but of what you're achieving. Watching that "amount saved" column grow - even slowly - can be deeply affirming.

It's also helpful to divide your costs into **essentials** and **electives**. Essentials are required for treatment: the procedure itself, medications, baseline monitoring. Electives may include things like genetic testing, embryo photos, or additional lab technology. Some electives are medically recommended. Others are optional, based on personal preference or clinic protocol. Knowing the difference can help you prioritise your spending without guilt.

It's tempting to throw everything into the "must have" category when your heart's on the line. But part of financial clarity is remembering that you're allowed to ask questions like: *Is this necessary for my specific case? Is there evidence this will improve my chances? Can it wait until later?*

A woman I worked with once asked her clinic about time-lapse embryo monitoring - an elective add-on that cost nearly £1,000. After reviewing the clinic's data, she realised it didn't significantly improve outcomes in her age group. She declined it, redirected that money to medication, and never regretted the decision. Her takeaway? *Saying no to something didn't mean I was saying no to my baby.*

The final layer of your fertility budget is perhaps the most powerful: **the flexibility column**. This is where you hold space for change. Because as much as we want to believe in neat timelines and stable numbers, IVF doesn't often work that way. Medications may need adjusting. A cycle might be postponed. A second round may become necessary. Flexibility is your cushion – your way of saying, *I knew this might happen, and I'm ready.*

Try to build in a small buffer – even £300–£500 – for those unexpected shifts. This doesn't have to be set aside all at once. It can grow slowly, alongside the rest of your savings. The goal is not to cover every possible detour. It's to reduce the shock when the route changes.

Some families also keep a small "emergency joy fund" within their budget – money for something comforting when things feel particularly heavy. It might go toward a dinner out after bad news, a massage before egg retrieval, or a weekend escape between cycles. This isn't indulgent. It's restorative. IVF can take over your whole emotional landscape. These small acts of care help you reclaim pieces of yourself along the way.

As your plan takes shape, revisit it regularly – not obsessively, but intentionally. Once a week. Once a month. After big appointments. You're not just watching numbers. You're tending to a living plan – one that reflects not just your finances, but your faith in what's possible.

Budgeting doesn't make IVF easy. But it does make it feel **less like chaos**. It puts a structure beneath your hope. It helps you make decisions you can live with. And it gives you the dignity of moving forward with your eyes open, your values intact, and your hand still on the wheel.

In the next section, we'll explore how to share the emotional load of budgeting - how to co-plan with your partner (if you have one), manage the mental labour of financial decisions, and keep space in your life for moments of joy.

There's a side of budgeting that no one really talks about - not the maths, not the money, but the *emotional management*. IVF doesn't just ask for your savings. It asks for your bandwidth, your energy, your attention, and, quite often, your sense of peace.

Even the most well-organised fertility budget can become a point of tension if the emotional labor behind it isn't acknowledged. Who's checking the spreadsheets? Who's making the difficult calls to insurance? Who's chasing pharmacy invoices, researching grants, or deciding whether to splurge on embryo glue?

In most relationships, especially in hetero partnerships, the weight of emotional and logistical labor often falls unequally. And when it comes to fertility, that imbalance can become magnified. It's not just about division of tasks - it's about how supported each person feels in a process that can so easily become overwhelming.

That's why one of the most important things you can do -

whether you're single or partnered – is to name and share the mental load of this journey. Start by identifying the roles and responsibilities that come with managing your fertility budget. These might include tracking payments, applying for support schemes, coordinating appointment logistics, or handling communication with the clinic. Then ask: *Who's doing what?* And more importantly: *Is it working?*

Some couples find it helpful to divide responsibilities based on strengths – maybe one person handles the numbers, while the other manages logistics or grant research. Others rotate roles monthly, or hold regular "budget check-ins" where both partners come to the table with updates and needs. It's less about perfect equality and more about mutual acknowledgement. Even a fifteen-minute conversation each week can create space for rebalancing.

One couple I supported created a standing Friday night ritual. They lit a candle, poured something they both enjoyed, and reviewed their budget. Sometimes they'd celebrate a win – a small saving or unexpected reimbursement. Sometimes they'd just sit quietly, admitting it felt hard. But always, they ended the conversation on the same side: *Us vs. the problem, not us vs. each other.*

If you're going through IVF alone, the emotional labor can feel doubly heavy. In this case, delegation doesn't have to mean partnership. Who else can help hold part of the load? A trusted friend who reviews invoices with you? A sibling who helps with clinic communication? A financial counselor who helps interpret dense insurance paperwork? You don't have to carry it all yourself. Sometimes sharing the burden starts with simply asking, *Would you sit with me while I sort this out?*

Just as important as shared responsibility is **emotional permission** - the freedom to say, *I need a break from thinking about this.* Budget fatigue is real. So is grief fatigue. You don't need to be endlessly productive or positive. In fact, rest is part of resilience. Building planned pauses into your process - even tiny ones - can help you return to decision-making with a clearer head and a steadier heart.

Create micro-boundaries around your IVF budget work. Maybe you only update your tracker on Sunday afternoons. Maybe you don't open billing emails at night. Maybe you designate one weekend a month as IVF-free - no appointments, no budgeting, no baby talk. These rituals of containment help you preserve your mental and emotional energy. You're not ignoring the process. You're protecting your capacity to *stay in it.*

Also, don't underestimate the value of ritualised comfort within the budgeting process. If managing money brings up fear or scarcity - and for many people it does - pair it with something soothing. Light a candle. Play calming music. Wrap yourself in a soft jumper. Drink something warm while you scan your receipts. These sensory anchors help remind your nervous system that you are safe - even in moments of stress.

And allow joy. Not in the "be grateful no matter what" kind of way, but in the small, defiant moments of reclaiming your life outside of spreadsheets and cycles. Build space into your budget for these things. A post-injection pastry. A favourite book. A surprise gift for yourself when you hit a savings goal. IVF is not all of you. You still get to live.

Above all, remember that the point of this budget is not perfection. It's not about executing a flawless plan or proving anything to anyone. The point is **protection** – protecting your heart, your relationships, your energy, and your agency. You are allowed to make decisions that make sense *for you*, even if they don't line up with someone else's timeline or treatment plan. Your budget should reflect your values – not just your balance sheet.

So as you look ahead, keep asking the questions that matter:

What do I need to feel supported?

What does my body need during this part of the process?

What's worth spending on – not because it guarantees success, but because it helps me feel like myself?

When you have a budget that makes room for those answers, you have more than a financial tool. You have a framework for moving forward – with clarity, with intention, and with care.

In the next chapter, we'll explore the many ways to increase your resources – from creative income strategies to community-based support – without burning out in the process.

5

Creative Income Strategies That Don't Burn You Out

"What if earning more didn't have to mean doing more?"

When you start talking about the cost of IVF, it's not long before someone brings up side hustles. "You could freelance! Sell things online! Start a business on Etsy!" But let's be honest - if you're already juggling a full-time job, hormone treatments, and the emotional intensity of fertility care, the last thing you need is pressure to become a productivity machine.

Still, there's often a very real gap between what treatment costs and what's currently available in your account. So this chapter is about **bridging that gap** - not with burnout, but with creativity, sustainability, and a deep respect for your energy. You don't need to "monetise your every moment." You just need options that work *with* your life, not against it.

The first step is to identify opportunities for **low-stress, flexible income** - the kind that slips into the margins of your week without demanding constant emotional output. This could be anything from tutoring in your area of expertise to offering voiceover recordings, selling digital downloads, or participating in paid surveys.

The trick is to look not just at what you *can* do, but what you're already doing – your skills, your rhythms, your natural flow – and see where small exchanges of value might exist. One woman I spoke to taught piano once a week to a neighbour's child. She didn't advertise it. She didn't try to scale it. But that one hour a week covered her acupuncture sessions and gave her a sense of gentle control over her budget.

Digital platforms also open doors for those needing flexibility. Websites like Fiverr, Upwork, or TaskRabbit can be useful for short, skill-based projects, whether it's proofreading, transcribing, graphic design, or tech support. But always check in with yourself: *Does this feel doable, or draining?* The goal isn't more hustle – it's intentional contribution.

Passive income is another underexplored pathway. Now, let's be clear: "passive" doesn't mean "instant." But if you already have something valuable – a design, a planner, a course, a skill – there are platforms that allow you to sell it repeatedly without constantly recreating it. Think: Canva templates, downloadable meal plans, guided meditations, photography presets, or niche digital products on Gumroad or Etsy. The creation takes effort up front, but once it's live, the maintenance is minimal.

If you're a maker or creator, selling physical items can be rewarding too – but tread carefully. Handmade products (candles, soaps, crochet, jewellery) can also lead to overwork. Ask yourself: *What's the minimum output that would still feel joyful?* Sometimes it's better to run a one-time pre-order than to open a full storefront. Boundaries keep passion from turning into pressure.

Beyond extra income, there's also value in **micro-optimisations** - subtle shifts in how your current money flows. For instance, check whether your employer offers fertility benefits or access to a Health Savings Account. You might also explore cashback credit cards (used responsibly), referral bonuses, or consolidating subscriptions. None of these changes will fund an entire cycle - but together, they ease friction. And reducing friction is a kind of gain, too.

Some families hold one-time fundraisers, like garage sales, bake sales, or silent auctions. Others create personal IVF fundraising pages through platforms like GoFundMe or PayPal Giving. This can feel deeply vulnerable, and only you can decide if that route aligns with your values. But if you do choose it, frame it with care: this isn't about asking for charity - it's about inviting your community to be part of something tender and hopeful. You'd be surprised how many people want to show up for you when given a chance.

There's also creative bartering. A friend of mine offered social media support to a small business in exchange for a few months of therapy. Another swapped tutoring hours for childcare. These aren't just budget wins - they're reminders that value doesn't always look like money, and that **community is part of the currency of care**.

What matters most in all of this is that your income strategies **support you, not drain you**. You're already doing something emotionally intense. Don't add a financial plan that feels like punishment. Instead, ask: *What feels light? What brings in a little ease? What supports the dream without swallowing the present?*

You are not lazy if you choose rest over extra hours. You are not less deserving because your income is fixed or limited. Worthiness isn't earned. IVF can make people feel like they have to prove how badly they want this – how hard they're willing to work, how much they're willing to sacrifice. But your value is not up for debate. You're already enough.

That's why this chapter isn't about squeezing more out of yourself. It's about finding more that fits – and giving yourself permission to do so gently.

Maximise What You Have

Sometimes, when the numbers don't seem to add up – when the gap between what you need and what you have feels too wide – the most grounding shift isn't trying to earn more. It's asking: *What am I already holding? And how can I use it differently?*

Maximising your current resources doesn't mean cutting joy or depriving yourself. It means opening up new possibilities with what's already in reach. This isn't about working harder. It's about thinking with care and flexibility – approaching your existing assets as allies in the fertility process.

One of the most powerful, underestimated resources you have is **your skillset**. Not just your formal qualifications, but the full inventory of what you know how to do – and what people naturally come to you for. Maybe you're the person who edits everyone's CVs. Or the one who bakes bread like it came from a patisserie. Or the friend who's always been able to fix a broken lamp with a YouTube tutorial and some clever thinking. These are not just hobbies. They're forms of quiet capital.

Start by writing down a list of your usable skills - things you're confident doing, or at least willing to offer in small doses. Then ask yourself: is there a simple, low-lift way to share this for value? Not necessarily money - though that's helpful - but barter, community exchange, or part-time pay. One woman I know offered Sunday meal prep sessions for busy new mums in her neighborhood. She wasn't trying to build a business. She just wanted to contribute, and it helped cover her acupuncture costs during IVF.

This mindset shift - from "I have nothing extra to give" to "I might already have something someone else needs" - is powerful. It returns a sense of agency that can so often feel lost when you're in a fertility journey shaped by medical jargon and financial overwhelm.

Another resource often overlooked is **your existing financial infrastructure** - the accounts, benefits, and systems you already use. Are you using them in the most supportive way? For example, check your bank for round-up savings tools, where purchases are rounded to the nearest pound and the difference is funneled into a savings pot. It sounds minor, but those incremental deposits can become meaningful over time - and require zero extra effort.

Some families set up automatic transfers to their fertility fund every payday - not large sums, but consistent ones. £25, £50, £75. The amount isn't the headline. The **habit** is. It creates a rhythm of contribution that steadily builds both funds and confidence.

Also, revisit your employer benefits. Many companies now offer **fertility-related coverage** - but don't always advertise it clearly. Look for wellness stipends, health savings accounts, or extended family leave options that can ease costs indirectly. One reader found out her company offered a £500 wellness benefit she could use toward counselling, which freed up funds for medication. Another learned that her corporate health insurance covered her fertility blood work even though IVF itself wasn't included.

If you're in a unionised job, check if there are negotiated benefits for reproductive care. Teachers, public servants, and NHS employees sometimes have access to support schemes through their unions that aren't broadly promoted. It's always worth asking - because even a partial coverage can shift your budget dramatically.

In your day-to-day life, small but intentional shifts in spending can also create meaningful room. This isn't about cutting everything joyful - it's about trimming the unnoticed excess that doesn't serve your values. For example, maybe you keep your morning coffee habit, because it brings you comfort on clinic days - but you cancel two streaming services you barely use. That's not sacrifice. That's **alignment**.

Go through one month of bank transactions and ask:

- What brought me real value or peace?
- What felt like autopilot?

- Where did my money go that I didn't even notice?

This practice isn't about judgment. It's about seeing clearly - and then making choices that feel more rooted in the version of you that's building a family.

Another underused resource: **your space**. Do you have a spare room, a garden plot, a driveway? These can sometimes be used creatively to generate short-term support without demanding much effort. I've known people who:

- Rented their parking space during events
- Let out their guest room for a week during peak holiday season
- Hosted small garden yoga classes
- Rented out a campervan or shed workspace temporarily

These ideas won't be right for everyone - and none of them are silver bullets. But when considered together, they paint a picture of potential. When you shift from thinking "I need to find money" to "I might already be holding value," the whole narrative changes.

Equally important is **social capital** - not in the networking sense, but in the deeply human sense. Who in your circle might want to help - and hasn't known how?

It's easy to assume we must carry everything quietly. IVF often brings with it a fierce desire to be self-reliant, to prove we're strong enough to manage this. But sharing your story – carefully, and with boundaries – can also open doors. Perhaps a friend's company has a generous fertility grant program. Perhaps someone's parent is a pharmacist who knows how to access discounted medication. Perhaps someone simply says, "I've been through this. I can help."

These aren't handouts. They're **pathways**. Fertility is so often portrayed as an individual battle – but in truth, it's a deeply communal experience. You're building a family. And families, by nature, are built on connection.

The courage to share – and the discernment to decide who to share with – can make all the difference.

Finally, don't underestimate the power of **celebrating small financial wins**. IVF can make you feel like everything hinges on thousands of pounds. But every £10 saved, every medication you found cheaper, every grant application you submitted – it matters. It reinforces the story that you *are* making progress, even when the journey feels slow.

One couple I know kept a visible savings tracker on their fridge. Every time they added to their fund – even £5 – they coloured in a block. That visual reminder was more than motivational. It was an emotional anchor. *We're getting there. Bit by bit.*

And that's the heartbeat of this section. You *are* getting there. Not through hustle, not through shame, but through intention, creativity, and self-respect. You're learning how to use what you have – your skills, your structure, your community – in a way that supports the future you're building.

Next, we'll explore ways to widen your financial circle even further – through funding options, grants, and structured support programs that can help shoulder the cost and reduce pressure on your monthly income.

Open the Circle - Grants, Loans, and Collective Support

For so many people on the fertility path, the challenge isn't just that IVF is expensive – it's that the costs arrive all at once, and often with little warning. You can plan, save, work extra hours, cut expenses, and still come up short. And it's here, in this difficult space between personal effort and reality, that external funding can change everything.

Yet many people don't know these resources exist – or they assume they won't qualify, or that applying is too overwhelming. That's understandable. When you're navigating ultrasounds and injections and emotional peaks and valleys, adding "find and apply for funding" to your list can feel like just one more impossible task.

But let me tell you something that many people only realise later: **you are allowed to ask for help.** You are allowed to lean on existing structures, programs, and communities that were built – quite literally – for people like you. Receiving support does not diminish your strength. In fact, accepting help often takes more courage than going it alone.

Let's start with grants. There are a growing number of nonprofit organisations that offer fertility grants, covering anything from medication to full IVF cycles. Some are country-specific, some are global. Some are based on financial need; others are open to anyone undergoing treatment. Many are designed to support marginalised groups: LGBTQ+ families, single parents, cancer survivors, or those facing medical infertility not covered by insurance.

Application processes vary, but most ask for a short personal statement, basic financial documentation, and proof of diagnosis or treatment plan. It can feel deeply vulnerable to put your story into words – but this act of storytelling can be empowering, too. One woman I worked with said that writing her grant essay was the first time she'd put her experience into language – and in doing so, she felt less alone.

A few well-regarded organisations to explore (note: readers should check for availability in their region):

- The Fertility Foundation
- Baby Quest Foundation
- The Hope for Fertility Foundation
- Access Fertility (UK)
- Parla or Tommy's (UK, often have pilot support programs)

Each year, these organisations help thousands of families begin treatment who otherwise wouldn't have access. Is the process competitive? Sometimes, yes. But the existence of these grants is a lifeline. And applying is always worth a try.

Then there's the question of **financing**. Fertility loans can feel risky – and in some cases, they are. But there are also structured payment plans, clinic-affiliated financing programs, and low-interest medical loans that can make treatment more accessible. The key here is clarity and caution.

Before taking out any loan:

- Ask your clinic if they partner with a specific lender or offer internal payment plans
- Read the fine print: interest rates, repayment terms, penalties
- Be realistic about your monthly repayment ability, especially if treatment doesn't work immediately
- Compare options: banks, credit unions, and fertility-specific lenders may all offer different terms

Some people also explore 0% interest credit cards or short-term family loans. These options aren't for everyone, and they should be weighed carefully - but for some, they offer a bridge between hope and affordability.

One of the most promising developments in recent years is the rise of **employer fertility benefits**. Companies are increasingly offering support for IVF, egg freezing, donor cycles, and surrogacy through health plans or fertility-focused benefit providers. If you're employed - particularly by a medium or large company - don't assume the answer is no. Ask your HR department directly, and ask for specifics.

A UK-based teacher I know discovered, to her surprise, that her employer offered partial reimbursement for fertility medication, even though the policy didn't mention IVF by name. Another couple found that the husband's workplace allowed £5,000 in family-building reimbursement annually, no questions asked. It's not always clearly communicated - but it's often there, quietly available for those who ask.

If your workplace offers nothing formal, you might consider **advocating**. There are now templates and guides available online for approaching HR about adding fertility benefits - and in many cases, it starts with one employee raising their voice.

Beyond structured programs, there's something quieter, but no less powerful: **community support**. This includes donation-based funds from churches, synagogues, or mosques; small business sponsorships; even friends or family pooling together to gift a portion of your treatment. You might feel hesitant to open that door. But again, support doesn't diminish your independence. It reinforces the truth that **you are not meant to do this alone**.

One woman I worked with shared her story at a community fundraiser and was gifted £1,200 from friends and neighbours. Another set up a private Facebook group for family members to follow their IVF journey and contribute small amounts as they were able. The contributions weren't enormous, but they were meaningful - and the emotional backing carried just as much weight as the money.

Some couples use registries - not just for baby items, but for fertility treatment itself. Websites like PlumFund or Gift of Parenthood allow people to create wish lists for medical procedures, counselling, travel for treatment, or post-treatment care. If asking for financial help feels strange, think of it this way: people love to celebrate the dream of a new life. Giving them the chance to help you build that dream is a gift in itself.

In all these scenarios - grants, loans, benefits, community - what matters most is that the support fits *you*. That it feels like a relief, not a burden. That it protects your dignity, your values, and your emotional bandwidth.

And that you remember: seeking help is not an act of failure. It's an act of faith - in your family, in your future, in the idea that sometimes, just sometimes, the world makes space for you to be held.

Next, we'll turn toward boundaries - because managing finances and fertility isn't just about what you say yes to. It's also about **knowing what to say no to**, and how to protect your mental and emotional space while navigating the unpredictable nature of IVF.

6

The Power of Boundaries: Saying No Without Guilt

The Invisible Cost of Saying Yes

There comes a moment in nearly every fertility journey where you feel pulled in a dozen different directions. Do another test. Try another supplement. Book a second opinion. Say yes to one more scan, one more work obligation, one more dinner invitation that requires smiling through someone else's pregnancy news. It's not just your money that feels spread thin – it's your attention, your energy, your emotional skin.

Boundaries are often framed as a way to "guard your time" or "say no more often," but here, in the landscape of IVF, they take on deeper meaning. Boundaries are not just walls to keep things out. They are **containers** – the structures that hold your hope, your rest, your clarity, and your sense of self when everything around you feels porous and demanding.

To begin building those containers, we must first recognise the hidden costs of unfiltered "yes." The ways that small, well-meaning agreements - saying yes to a family gathering, agreeing to work overtime, responding to every well-intentioned message - can erode your inner space over time. Every yes comes from somewhere. Every yes has a cost. And when you're in the midst of fertility treatment, your margins are already razor-thin.

Start by noticing what I call *the invisible transaction* - the agreements you make without realising they're happening. Saying yes to a friend's baby shower, for example, might seem kind and expected. But underneath, it may cost you: emotional regulation, the energy to self-soothe afterward, a full day of your limited social fuel. Or consider agreeing to take on a big project at work because you don't want to seem unreliable - even though your mind is already split between clinic calendars and medication tracking.

None of these costs show up on a budget spreadsheet. But they are *real*. And when they go unacknowledged, they accumulate. What starts as a trickle - "I'll just say yes this one time" - becomes a flood of depletion. That depletion shows up everywhere: reduced patience, anxiety spirals, poor sleep, decision fatigue. It makes budgeting harder. It makes conversations more fraught. It chips away at your sense of control.

So the first step is simply to name the leak. Ask yourself:

- What am I currently saying yes to that feels automatic, rather than intentional?

- Which of these yeses leaves me feeling heavier, not lighter?
- If I didn't feel guilty or obligated, what would I decline?

You don't have to change anything yet. Just see it. Seeing the invisible transaction gives you the power to renegotiate it.

Once you begin noticing these patterns, it becomes easier to sort them. Not every yes is problematic. Some yeses are life-giving - yes to a friend who truly understands, yes to a gentle yoga class, yes to a Friday night film that helps you feel normal again. The goal isn't to eliminate all yeses - it's to **get deliberate about them**.

A woman I supported once told me she used to say yes to every social event out of fear she'd miss out - or worse, be forgotten. But after three cycles of IVF, she started asking herself: *Will this replenish me, or require repair?* If the answer was repair - if she knew she'd need days to emotionally recover afterward - she gave herself permission to opt out. Not rudely. Not dramatically. Just honestly.

And here's the thing: boundaries don't need to be hard-edged to be effective. They can be soft and loving. They can be kind. Saying "I can't make it, but I'm thinking of you" is still a boundary. So is "I'm not up for a call right now, but I appreciate you checking in." You don't need to over-explain. You don't need to make up reasons. *You are allowed to choose quiet, rest, and privacy.*

It also helps to create **default scripts** - gentle phrases you can reach for when caught off guard. These become your anchors in moments of discomfort:

- "That's not something I can commit to right now, but thank you for understanding."
- "I'm focusing on my health at the moment, so I'm keeping things pretty low-key."
- "That's not a good fit for me right now, but I really appreciate you thinking of me."

These scripts reduce the emotional labour of boundary-setting in real time. They give you language when your heart is already tired.

Boundaries also belong in the financial space. One of the most common pressure points during IVF is feeling like you *should* be doing or buying more. The ads for supplements. The "must-have" testing add-ons. The clinic upsells. The gentle suggestions from others that *maybe* you should consider just one more intervention.

Here's the truth: just because something is available - or even recommended - doesn't mean it's right for you. Your boundary might be financial ("We're not going to add another £2,000 test unless it's truly necessary"). Or emotional ("We're not going to spend another six weeks chasing conflicting second opinions"). Your values get to shape your plan.

That's not recklessness. That's discernment. One of the strongest, most protective boundaries you can hold is the one that says: *We will not let fear run the show.*

This doesn't mean you're closed to options. It means you

evaluate them from a place of groundedness, not panic. You weigh them against your specific case, your budget, your energy – and you choose from there.

Boundaries are also essential in your conversations. IVF brings out advice – sometimes from kind places, sometimes from deep misunderstanding. If someone keeps offering unsolicited tips, or if every conversation turns toward their own experience, you're allowed to say: "I appreciate you wanting to help. What I really need right now is just someone to listen."

One client of mine created a simple visual for family visits – a candle on the kitchen table. If it was lit, it meant: *No fertility talk today.* Everyone respected it. It gave her a way to signal her limits without constant explanation.

That's what good boundaries do – they **protect without punishing**. They allow relationships to continue, safely. They allow you to rest inside yourself. They make space for IVF to be part of your life, *not your whole life*.

In the next section, we'll talk about how to identify your personal boundary triggers – and how to create sustainable systems around work, communication, time, and self-care that serve your mental health during treatment.

Your Triggers, Your Terms

Everyone carries their own boundary blueprint. Some of us are wired to avoid conflict. Others feel guilty the moment we say no.

Some grew up in homes where being helpful was survival. Some were told that "selfish" was the worst thing you could be. And when something as raw and tender as fertility treatment enters the picture, those old wiring patterns light up like a switchboard.

This section is about recognising those patterns - not with judgment, but with care. Because once you understand your emotional triggers around boundary-setting, you can start to set terms that actually work for *you*. Not the version of you that people expect. The real you. The you who's holding so much already.

Let's begin with a simple but powerful idea: *you are allowed to have limits, even if others don't understand them.*

That includes financial limits. Social limits. Time limits. Emotional limits. IVF asks a lot - and the world around you often expects you to keep showing up as if nothing's changed. That's not only unrealistic - it's damaging. Pretending to be okay to keep others comfortable is a silent energy leak. And energy, right now, is your most precious currency.

So how do you identify your personal triggers? Look for the moments that make you feel:

- Drained before something even begins
- Flooded with guilt after you say no
- Resentful for saying yes
- Like you need to rehearse your response over and over
- Responsible for someone else's disappointment

These emotional cues are your compass. They don't mean

you're failing. They mean you're on the edge of a boundary - one that probably hasn't been named yet.

Let's take an example. Suppose every time your sibling asks how IVF is going, you feel a mix of anxiety and pressure - because you know they'll ask, "Have you tried X?" or "Maybe it's stress?" and you'll end up justifying choices you barely have the energy to make.

That's a boundary moment. You're being asked to perform emotional clarity at a time when what you really need is compassion. In that case, your term might sound like:

- "I'd love to update you when I have something I feel ready to share."
- "I appreciate you asking - right now I'm trying to keep a little space around it."

Notice the tone: respectful, but protective. Honest, but not defensive.

This is what boundary work really looks like. Not confrontation, but calibration.

It's also helpful to build **boundary systems** - structures that hold your boundaries for you so you're not constantly doing emotional heavy lifting. These systems can be as simple as:

- A shared calendar with "quiet days" blocked out
- A prewritten email template to respond to treatment inquiries
- A budgeting plan that includes "non-negotiable" rest or recovery costs

- Setting up auto-replies on days when you're processing difficult news

You shouldn't need to *earn* rest. You shouldn't need to explain why you're unavailable after an injection-heavy week. Let your systems do the work. The fewer moments you have to justify yourself, the more energy you reclaim.

One woman I worked with set up a colour-coded calendar system with her partner. Red days = retrievals or emotionally hard milestones. Yellow days = prep and admin. Green days = no IVF talk unless invited. It wasn't rigid - it was responsive. And most importantly, it made her feel seen.

You might also find it useful to create a **boundary mantra** - something short you can return to when self-doubt creeps in. Some examples:

- "My peace is worth protecting."
- "Saying no now makes space for yes later."
- "I'm allowed to disappoint others to take care of myself."
- "This season requires softness, not performance."

A mantra isn't a magic fix. But it *anchors* you. It gives your nervous system a hand to hold when the old guilt stories show up.

Another important area to establish boundaries is **online**. The fertility space on social media can be a gift - full of shared wisdom, solidarity, and support. But it can also become overwhelming. Comparison, unsolicited advice, and toxic positivity are real risks.

If you find that scrolling leaves you feeling more anxious than connected, that's a boundary signal. You're allowed to mute or unfollow, even if someone means well. You're allowed to log off. You're allowed to protect your timeline like you'd protect a nursery: tenderly, intentionally, with love.

This is especially true if your feed is filled with pregnancy announcements or miracle stories. There's nothing wrong with those moments. But if they sting – if they pull your focus away from your own process – you have every right to step back. One client of mine created a "fertility-only" Instagram account, followed just a few supportive voices, and let her main feed go quiet. She said it was the best thing she did for her mental health.

Boundaries are also a financial tool. Saying no to unnecessary treatments, declining upsells, choosing not to pursue a fourth opinion when your heart says stop – these are valid, powerful decisions. One couple I supported decided not to pursue a pricey ERA test after reading the evidence and discussing it with a trusted provider. They used the funds instead for counselling and an extended holiday before their final round. They didn't regret it.

This is the heart of what boundaries offer: *alignment*. When your external choices reflect your internal needs, you feel steadier. You stop chasing a finish line set by someone else. You return to yourself.

You get to say: This is what I need right now. Not forever. Just now. You get to change your mind. You get to hold your process gently – not because you're fragile, but because you are valuable.

And as you move through this chapter, I want you to remember that boundaries are not a rejection of others. They are an **affirmation of your own wholeness**. They are a way of saying, "I matter, too."

In the final part of this chapter, we'll look at boundaries as *community care* – how they strengthen partnerships, reduce resentment, and create space for real connection in a season that can feel lonely and full of emotional landmines.

Boundaries as a Form of Connection

We often think of boundaries as barriers. Something you put up to keep people out. But in the context of IVF – a journey that's intensely vulnerable, often isolating, and financially fraught – boundaries are not walls. They are *bridges*. They allow you to stay close without becoming overwhelmed. They allow others to support you without overstepping. And most of all, they allow you to be *honest*.

Let's begin with the place where most boundary work gets tested first: **your partnership**.

Whether you're navigating IVF with a spouse, a co-parent, or a chosen partner – or even if you're going it alone with a close friend or sibling walking beside you – this is where emotional load meets daily logistics. Conversations around money, timing, medical decisions, and hope (or fear) can easily tip into tension.

When there's no clear boundary between *your thoughts* and

their reactions, misunderstandings breed. One person might spiral into research mode, booking second opinions and spreadsheets. The other may go silent, overwhelmed and shut down. Without boundaries, we interpret these differences as lack of care – when in truth, they're just different coping strategies.

One of the most grounding tools you can use here is a **check-in ritual**. Set aside 10–15 minutes once or twice a week to talk, without distractions, about where you're both at. Not to make decisions. Not to fix each other. Just to speak and listen.

You might ask:

- What's feeling most tender this week?
- What's one decision we need to make together soon?
- What's one thing we could each let go of?

Creating space for these conversations *on purpose* means they're less likely to erupt in moments of stress. And within them, it's okay – necessary, even – to say, "I need a break from fertility talk today," or "I need some reassurance before we make this payment." These are boundaries. And when voiced gently and clearly, they invite closeness, not conflict.

I once supported a couple who, after their second failed round, started clashing about every small financial choice – dinner out, clothing, even petrol. Underneath it all was grief. They weren't really fighting about money. They were both just scared. When they began doing weekly budget reviews together with a "no-blame" rule, the tension eased. Their boundary wasn't financial – it was emotional: "We'll speak to each other as teammates, not opponents."

This is the connective power of boundaries. They create **a shared language of care**.

Outside of the home, boundaries with extended family and friends can be trickier. People often mean well, but say things that sting: "Just relax and it'll happen." "Why not adopt?" "You're young - you've got time." These comments come from discomfort, not malice - but they still hurt.

Setting a boundary here might sound like:

- "Thanks for caring. Right now we're being careful about what conversations we have around treatment."
- "We'd love your support, and what helps most is just listening, not problem-solving."
- "This is a hard season, and we're trying to keep our circle small right now."

You don't need to provide your full fertility history. You don't need to educate everyone. You just need to protect your peace. And the people who love you - really love you - will adapt.

One woman told me she sent a group email to her close family saying, "We're in the middle of IVF. We don't know what's going to happen. We're scared. Please don't ask for updates unless we offer them. Your love means more than your questions." Not everyone got it right. But many did. And the relief she felt in finally naming her needs was immense.

Sometimes, you'll encounter resistance - people who push back, accuse you of being distant, or take your boundaries personally. That's not a sign you're doing it wrong. That's a sign they're used to you overextending. Don't let their discomfort dislodge your clarity. You are allowed to change the rules of engagement - especially when the stakes are this high.

Let's not forget workplace boundaries. Many people undergoing IVF still work full time - often in environments that aren't fertility-aware. Whether or not you disclose your treatment is entirely up to you. But whatever you choose, you can set professional boundaries that protect your energy and privacy.

Examples include:

- Blocking out buffer time before and after appointments
- Saying no to extra responsibilities during high-intensity treatment windows
- Letting a trusted manager or colleague know you may need flexible hours, without disclosing every detail
- Taking mental health days when needed - they are just as valid as physical sick days

One client created a colour-coded shared calendar at work with only one label: "Unavailable." It was her quiet way of holding space for herself - and it worked.

In addition, boundaries around *technology* can make a world of difference. Set screen time limits. Designate "no-fertility zones" (the dinner table, your bedroom, Sunday mornings).

Turn off alerts for fertility apps if they spike anxiety. It's okay to take a full weekend away from research and results.

This helps you stay *present* - not permanently, but often enough to remember there is life happening alongside the waiting. Laughter. Music. Rain. People who love you.

Ultimately, boundaries aren't about pushing the world away. They're about **building the conditions for real connection**- the kind that doesn't deplete or demand, but restores.

And that's what you deserve: to feel held, seen, and supported. Not just by others, but by the systems you create. The choices you make. The quiet decisions you honour within yourself.

As we move into the next chapter, we'll talk about navigating the emotional rollercoaster of waiting - with practical tools for managing uncertainty, anxiety, and the constant pull of "what if?"

Because alongside money, boundaries, and planning... is the heart of it all: *hope, delayed.*

7

The Waiting Room: Coping with Delays, Disappointment, and the Unknown

The Space Between the News

There is a peculiar ache that settles in during IVF. It's not the procedures or the pills. It's the waiting. The endless waiting. Waiting for your period. Waiting to start. Waiting for a phone call. Waiting for a result that could change your entire life in the space of three words.

People will tell you to "just stay busy." But busyness doesn't dissolve the tension. It buries it. And when it resurfaces – which it always does – it brings with it all the anxiety that was never given space to breathe.

This is the *emotional economy* of fertility treatment. So much of your time is spent in the unknown. Not actively doing anything – just existing in the shadow of a possibility.

And that space – the space between the news – can become

suffocating if we don't learn how to meet it with tenderness, structure, and permission to feel.

Let's begin here: **waiting is not doing nothing.** It is a psychological load. A full-time mental job. It uses your imagination, your vigilance, your emotional resilience. So if you feel exhausted during a "quiet" week where nothing is scheduled, there's a reason.

One woman told me, "I felt more tired waiting for my beta results than I did after egg retrieval." That's the reality of prolonged emotional uncertainty. It mimics grief. It activates fear. And it's worsened by the feeling that everyone else is moving forward while you're standing still.

So how do we live well in this space?

The first shift is learning to name it - *not as a failure, but as a phase.* This isn't you stalling. This is a stage in the journey. Like winter in the natural cycle - bare branches, quiet soil, but still full of life underneath. Dormancy is not death. And just because something isn't visible doesn't mean it isn't changing you.

There are three kinds of waiting that most IVF patients encounter:

1. **Short-term medical waiting** - test results, hormone levels, embryo viability
2. **Treatment delays** - clinic backlogs, unexpected findings, illness
3. **Life-stage limbo** - waiting for a partner's readiness, a job to stabilise, a savings goal to be met

Each of these kinds of waiting brings its own texture. The sharp, anxious pulse of a two-week wait. The dull drag of postponed cycles. The ache of having everything ready – except the green light.

And here's the hard part: we don't control the clock.

So instead, we build **coping scaffolds**. Temporary structures that support us through the weight of time.

The first scaffold is **ritual**. Unlike routine, which is practical, ritual is emotional. It transforms repetition into meaning. Lighting a candle after an injection. Journaling each morning with a fertility mantra. Taking a walk at the same time each day to steady your breath. Rituals anchor you. They give shape to the formless.

One woman I supported had a jar filled with coloured stones. Every day she waited, she added one. When her treatment ended – successfully or not – she planned to bury them in the garden. "I want to remember this time as something I lived through," she said. "Not just something I tried to get over."

The second scaffold is **containment**. It's a gentle way of saying: not all emotions need to spill everywhere, all the time. Containment means choosing where and when to feel. Giving yourself full permission to cry – but not letting panic take the wheel during work meetings. It means creating emotional "containers" where you can safely unload.

This could be:

- Talking to a therapist or coach once a week
- Writing down your fears before bed
- Designating 10 minutes a day for a "worry release" journal entry
- Joining a closed, moderated online community where you feel seen

Containment isn't about denying pain. It's about *protecting your energy* so you can survive this process intact.

The third scaffold is **micro-choice** - the practice of choosing small things, every day, to reclaim agency in an uncontrollable system. You can't decide when implantation occurs. But you can decide:

- What to eat for breakfast
- Which book to read
- Whether to share this part of the journey with someone new
- How to soothe your nervous system today

These tiny choices keep your identity alive. You are not only a patient. You are a person, still building a life.

And speaking of life - there's something quietly radical about allowing joy into this waiting. You don't have to postpone your happiness until you know the outcome. You can let yourself laugh, travel, buy flowers, paint, kiss, dance. Not as distraction. But as *nourishment*.

Joy does not betray your longing. It *buoys* it.

That's the paradox of IVF waiting: it asks you to live in two places at once - the not-yet, and the right-now. And you're allowed to honour both.

As we move into the next section, we'll explore what happens when waiting turns into disappointment - and how to walk through grief, plan the next step, or pause entirely without losing yourself in the process.

When Hope Hurts - Moving Through Disappointment

No matter how well you prepare - financially, emotionally, logistically - there's no insurance policy against heartbreak in IVF. Even with the best doctors. Even with the most diligent planning. Sometimes the embryo doesn't implant. Sometimes the cycle gets cancelled. Sometimes the test comes back with news that makes your stomach fall.

And when it happens - when the thing you hoped for doesn't come - the world doesn't pause. Emails keep arriving. Bills keep showing up. People keep texting you things like "Any updates?" without realising those words land like bricks.

This section is for that moment. The moment after. The quiet devastation of a no.

Disappointment after IVF isn't just sadness. It's layered. It's sadness braided with exhaustion, frustration, guilt, anger, and sometimes even shame. It can make you question your choices, your body, your instincts. It can flatten everything you'd built your days around.

One woman I supported said, "I didn't just lose a cycle. I lost the whole scaffolding of the next three months. The vision I had. The timeline I'd built in my head."

Disappointment here is not abstract. It's time, money, energy, and hope – all seemingly gone in an instant.

So what do you *do* when your heart breaks but the world doesn't stop?

The first thing is simple: **don't rush yourself out of it.** Our culture – even the fertility world – tends to skip over this part. The "Try again!" messages. The inspirational quotes. The push to reframe, to move on, to stay positive.

But disappointment needs room. It needs to breathe. Grief, when ignored, doesn't shrink. It buries. And when buried, it resurfaces in anxiety, burnout, numbness, or resentment.

You are allowed to feel it all. You are allowed to lie on the bathroom floor and weep. You are allowed to cancel dinner plans and say, "I'm not okay." You are allowed to not be inspiring right now.

Grieving a failed round or a cancelled cycle doesn't mean you've lost faith. It means you're *human*.

Give your grief a name. Write it out. Tell someone. Say: "I am mourning this specific hope." Speak it. Let it be real.

But grief doesn't live alone. It always has companions. Often, **shame** walks right behind it – whispering things like "Maybe I waited too long," or "I should have done another test," or "Why can't I just be grateful for what I have?"

Shame lies. It tells you the outcome was a personal failure. But IVF – and fertility itself – is a biological process with too many variables to control. You cannot outwork or out-worry it into success.

If you're experiencing that shame spiral, try this:

- Write down the voices in your head
- Ask: Would I say these things to a friend in my shoes?
- Cross out any sentence that is unkind or untrue
- Replace it with one compassionate truth, like "I did the best I could with the information I had" or "I am worthy, regardless of the outcome"

Over time, that becomes your emotional baseline. Not blame. But compassion.

When you're ready – and only when you're ready – you can begin to think about *what comes next.*

For some, it's trying again. For others, it's pausing to rest. For some, it's reevaluating entirely: Do we want to pursue another round? Is this the right clinic? Do we need a second opinion? Do we need to change course?

All of these are valid. And none should be made in haste. Especially not in the immediate aftermath of loss.

One couple I knew set a 30-day rule: no new decisions about treatment for one month after a failed round. Instead, they focused on eating well, going for walks, reconnecting with friends, and sleeping without alarms. At the end of the month, they revisited their options with clearer heads and steadier hearts.

If you do choose to pause, know this: *pausing is not quitting.* It's recovery. It's wisdom. It's the space needed for your body, mind, and finances to reset. And often, it leads to better decisions.

You can also use this time to gather new information. Maybe schedule a review with your clinic. Maybe consult a fertility counsellor to help you process. Maybe explore a second opinion or alternative pathway, without committing yet. Learning doesn't have to equal action. Sometimes, it just helps you feel a little more in control.

Finally, this is the moment when you need your people - but only the ones who make space, not noise. The ones who ask "How are you?" and really want to hear the answer. The ones who don't try to fix or minimise.

One woman I worked with had a friend who simply texted, "Here if you want to scream, cry, or just sit in silence." That text meant more than all the "you'll get there!" messages combined.

If you don't have someone like that right now, consider a support group, a therapist, or an online circle. There are spaces - quiet, non-judgmental spaces - that exist just for this part of the journey. You are not alone.

As we move into the next section, we'll explore ways to hold on to hope - not in the blind, forced-positivity way, but in the rooted, grounded, we're-still-here way. Because hope, even when bruised, is still a powerful companion. And it deserves a place beside your grief, not in place of it.

A Steadier Kind of Hope

After a setback - whether it's a failed cycle, a postponement, or a conversation that didn't go the way you needed - hope can start to feel like a risky emotion. Too bright, too exposed. A thing you've dared to carry once before, only to watch it disappear in a flash of bad news or closed options. And yet, the desire to hope doesn't vanish. It lingers. Quietly. Sometimes guiltily. It waits for permission to return, to be held again without fear.

This section is about welcoming that hope back in - not the wide-eyed, all-or-nothing kind, but a steadier, slower, deeply rooted form of hope. The kind that coexists with uncertainty. The kind that breathes even when plans change.

One of the misconceptions around hope in the IVF world is that it has to be big and unwavering to be "real." But in truth, the most sustainable hope is often gentle and flexible. It adapts. It doesn't insist on one outcome. It says, "I still believe good things are possible - even if I don't know when or how they'll come."

This kind of hope begins not with promises, but with **presence**. It starts by acknowledging where you are - not skipping over the hard parts, but allowing them to sit alongside your longing. One woman I worked with once told me, "After our third loss, I stopped hoping for a baby. But I started hoping for mornings that didn't begin in tears. That was my way back in."

That shift - from outcome-focused to experience-focused - is the gateway to realistic hope. When you allow yourself to hope for rest, clarity, or even just a better day, you reclaim a sense of power. You're not waiting for the stars to align. You're tending to the ground beneath your feet.

A helpful practice here is *redefining your wins*. The fertility world often measures success in narrow terms: positive pregnancy tests, heartbeats on a scan, birth announcements. But those are only one part of the story. There are so many other kinds of progress that matter.

Maybe you advocated for yourself at your last clinic appointment. Maybe you saved enough to cover the next cycle without debt. Maybe you took a week off social media and felt your anxiety lessen. These are milestones. They may not get shared in glossy highlight reels, but they are signs of growth, strength, and clarity.

And when you track these small but significant shifts, you remind yourself that you're not stuck - you're evolving. Even now. Even in waiting.

Another way to nurture this steadier hope is to **revisit your why**. When the process feels long and hard, it's easy to lose sight of the reasons you began. Not just the dream of parenthood, but the values behind it. What kind of life are you trying to build? What kind of parent do you hope to be - not someday, but in how you show up for yourself now?

Sometimes reconnecting with your why brings new perspective. A couple I knew were deep into treatment and unsure whether to continue. They paused and asked themselves, "What would this child learn from watching us go through this?" That single question shifted their next steps. It wasn't about pushing through at all costs - it was about modelling care, resilience, and intentionality.

In practical terms, rebuilding hope also means creating moments of **emotional replenishment**. This isn't toxic positivity. This is strategic softness. You need joy. Not in large doses, necessarily, but regularly. Planned joy. Scheduled lightness. It might be a playlist that lifts your mood, a weekend with friends who don't talk about fertility, a trip to the ocean, or a quiet morning with no plans and no pressure.

These pockets of joy are not indulgent – they're **protective**. They help fortify your nervous system. They remind you that you are still a person, still deserving of beauty and connection and peace.

It can also help to create a hope journal – not a vision board or a rigid list of goals, but a gentle space where you record signs of movement, moments of resilience, and quotes or memories that remind you who you are. One page might read, "I asked for what I needed." Another might hold a photo of the walk you took after getting hard news. Over time, this becomes a living document of your courage. A private reminder that hope has many faces – and you've worn more of them than you think.

And then there's community. Nothing steadies hope like knowing you're not alone. When you hear someone else's story – not the highlight reel, but the full, human, messy truth – it can widen the edges of your own belief. Not in a comparison sense, but in a recognition: *they made it through. I can, too.*

If you feel isolated, try seeking out fertility support groups, virtual meetups, or even personal blogs and memoirs from those who've walked this road. Choose carefully – protect your boundaries – but know that shared experience is one of the most powerful reminders that hope is not foolish. It's human.

And finally, give yourself permission to hold hope lightly. You don't have to clutch it. You don't have to perform it. Some days, hope may simply be the fact that you got up, made tea, and sent an email to your clinic. That's enough.

Hope isn't a mood. It's a muscle. It can be rebuilt. And it will look different at every stage of your journey. The goal isn't to always feel hopeful - it's to stay open to hope's return, again and again, in new and unexpected forms.

As we close this chapter, we move from the emotional territory of waiting to the logistical terrain of navigating the medical system itself. In Chapter Seven, we'll walk through how to be your own advocate - asking the right questions, pushing past confusing jargon, and making sure you're heard, understood, and treated with the dignity every patient deserves.

8

The Informed Patient: How to Advocate for Yourself Without Burning Out

Decoding the Medical Maze

There's a moment in almost every fertility journey when you find yourself sitting across from a specialist, nodding politely, while a wave of acronyms, protocols, and probabilities floods the room. You're trying to absorb it all - the hormone levels, the treatment plans, the percentages - but somewhere between "AMH" and "blastocyst," your brain freezes. You leave the clinic with a stack of printouts, a tentative timeline, and a sinking feeling: *I'm not sure what just happened - and I'm not sure what comes next.*

This is the medical maze. It's real. It's overwhelming. And it's one of the most disempowering parts of the fertility process - not because patients aren't smart or capable, but because the system often forgets that this is all brand new to you.

This section is about reclaiming your power in that space. Not by becoming a fertility expert overnight – but by becoming an *informed*, *confident*, and *centered* participant in your own care.

First, let's name the problem plainly: the fertility industry can feel intimidating. Even when your provider is kind, the culture around IVF is built on technical jargon and unspoken hierarchies. You might feel like you're "not allowed" to ask certain questions. Or that if you don't agree with the suggested plan immediately, you're being difficult. Add to that the emotional stakes – your time, money, and dreams – and it's easy to feel like you have no choice but to go along.

But you do have choices. And the most important tool you have is *clarity*.

One of the most effective ways to gain clarity in a medical setting is to shift your mindset before the appointment. Instead of walking in as a passive recipient of information, you go in as a **partner in decision-making**. That simple reframe changes everything.

You're not just there to be told what to do. You're there to collaborate. To ask. To push for what you need to feel safe, seen, and understood.

That begins with preparation. Before each appointment – even virtual ones – take fifteen minutes to ground yourself:

- Write down three questions you want answered
- Highlight any terms you didn't understand from a previous visit
- Note anything that felt rushed, unclear, or overwhelming

- Remind yourself that asking questions is not rude – it's responsible

Many patients feel like they have to "perform" being agreeable to be taken seriously. But a respectful question is not confrontation – it's self-advocacy. And you are allowed to be thorough.

Here's a truth that gets overlooked: **clinics work for you**. You are their patient, but also their client. You are making medical decisions that will shape your finances, your body, your emotions, and your family. That gives you every right to ask:

- What are the alternatives to this procedure?
- What's the evidence behind this protocol?
- Are there additional costs I should be aware of?
- Can you walk me through the risks and benefits in plain language?

If the answers are unclear, ask again. Ask for written information. Ask to delay the decision if you need time to think. This is not about being combative – it's about creating *informed consent*. You deserve full transparency before making any medical or financial commitment.

It can help to bring a second person to appointments, especially those where decisions are likely to be made. They don't have to be your partner – a friend, sibling, or even a doula trained in fertility advocacy can be invaluable. Their job isn't to speak for you but to help you stay grounded, take notes, and remind you of your priorities if the conversation veers off course.

And yes, bring a notebook. Or use your phone's voice recorder (with permission). Don't rely on memory - your nervous system is likely operating on high alert. Write things down so you can revisit them later when the adrenaline has eased and your thoughts have settled.

Here's something that often gets missed: **you are allowed to change providers.** Just because you've started with one clinic doesn't mean you're stuck there. If something doesn't feel right - if communication is poor, if you feel dismissed, if your questions go unanswered - you are allowed to seek a second opinion or transfer care. You are not being disloyal. You are protecting your process.

I once worked with a client who changed clinics mid-treatment, not because her previous provider had made any clinical mistakes, but because the emotional environment was cold. She said, "I needed someone to remember I was a person, not just a set of hormone levels." Her second clinic didn't have better statistics - but the experience felt entirely different. And her mental health improved overnight.

Sometimes, advocating for yourself means pushing back on unnecessary interventions. The fertility industry is full of optional (and often expensive) add-ons. Some may be beneficial in specific cases, but many are offered routinely without strong evidence. If you're presented with a new test, supplement, or treatment:

- Ask: Is this essential for my case?
- Ask: Will this improve my outcome - or just give us more data?

- Ask: What does the current research say?

You do not need to say yes on the spot. A wise patient once told me, "If it's worth doing, it's worth sleeping on."

This section also wouldn't be complete without mentioning **language**. The words clinicians use matter. If you've been told your "eggs are old," or that "you waited too long," or if you've been spoken to in ways that feel shaming or dismissive, please know: that is not acceptable. And it's not your fault. Medical language should never harm. If it does, that's a cue to speak up – or step away.

Lastly, being your own advocate doesn't mean doing everything alone. It means creating a system of support around you – people, tools, resources – that help you show up as your own best ally. You don't have to know everything. You just need to know *enough to feel steady.*

In the next section, we'll explore how to build this support system more intentionally – not just emotionally, but logistically, so that the decisions you make about your care are never made in isolation.

Building Your Support System - People, Tools, and Practical Help

In the world of IVF, you're often cast in the role of lead actor, stage manager, director, and lighting crew - all at once. You're expected to remember every appointment, track your own data, process complex emotions, and manage a constantly shifting budget. And while much of the journey is indeed personal, it was never meant to be walked alone.

Every strong advocate needs a support structure. This doesn't mean you need an army of experts or a cheering squad at every turn. It means creating a *reliable, responsive system* that keeps you from crumbling under the weight of it all - especially when emotions are high and clarity is hard to reach.

Start with **your inner circle** - the people you trust most. This might include your partner, a close friend, a parent, or a sibling. The role of your inner circle is not to understand every nuance of your treatment plan, but to be emotionally safe and practically supportive. People who can hold space for your frustration without judgment. People who ask "Do you want to vent, or problem-solve?" before jumping in. People who check in not just for updates, but for *you.*

If you have a partner, it's crucial to clarify roles. Fertility treatment has a way of magnifying everyday imbalances. Maybe one of you is the researcher, and the other is the feeler. Maybe one manages logistics, and the other shuts down in overwhelm. These patterns are normal - but if left unspoken, they can breed resentment.

Have a weekly sit-down to check in on:

- What decisions need to be made this week
- How each of you is coping emotionally
- Any practical tasks that can be redistributed or delayed

Even a ten-minute conversation can prevent misunderstandings and help you feel like a team again - even when the path is unclear.

Beyond your closest people, consider your **extended circle**. These are the people who may not walk with you every day, but whose contributions are meaningful. This might include:

- A therapist with fertility experience
- A financial planner familiar with medical costs
- A coach, mentor, or support group facilitator
- A trusted friend who's been through IVF and can offer honest reflections without prescribing

If therapy isn't financially accessible right now, look for support groups run by fertility clinics or nonprofits. Many offer low-cost or free virtual options. Peer-led groups can also be powerful - not for medical advice, but for shared emotional resonance.

One woman I worked with joined a weekly "quiet circle" - a virtual gathering where participants simply shared how their week was going without fixing or comparing. That hour became the one place where she didn't have to pretend she was okay. That's the power of soft structure: it doesn't solve your grief, but it holds it with you.

Next, think about **logistical support** - the tools and practices that make the day-to-day smoother. You don't need an elaborate system. Just enough scaffolding to give your brain some breathing room. Consider:

- A dedicated fertility calendar (digital or physical) for appointments, medication reminders, and budgeting deadlines
- A shared Google Drive or folder for storing clinic documents, invoices, lab results, and treatment notes
- A "question bank" where you jot down things to ask at upcoming appointments
- A simple checklist of your current cycle's steps, taped to the fridge or saved to your phone

These aren't just organisational tools - they're *emotional stabilisers.* They reduce decision fatigue and help you see progress, even on days when everything feels uncertain.

If you're a visual thinker, apps like Fertility Friend, Ovia, or Clue can help track symptoms and treatments. But beware of overtracking. Sometimes, too much data can heighten anxiety. Choose tools that clarify, not clutter. And if a tool stops serving you, let it go.

Finally, let's talk about **energy management**. Being your own advocate takes mental and emotional energy - and that energy is not unlimited. Protect it by outsourcing when you can, even in small ways:

- Automate bill payments where possible
- Ask a friend to help you compile questions for an upcoming consult
- Delegate a household task or two during treatment weeks
- Set a boundary around which days you'll engage with fertility research (e.g. "I don't Google after 8 p.m.")

Think of this as *practical self-advocacy*. You don't have to push through alone to prove your strength. You can build a network – even a quiet one – that reinforces your resilience and reminds you that you're not navigating this maze without a map or a hand to hold.

In the next section, we'll take this one step further – exploring how to handle difficult conversations with your care team when you feel dismissed, ignored, or uncertain. Because being an informed patient doesn't mean everything goes smoothly – it means you know how to respond when it doesn't.

What to Do When You're Not Being Heard

No matter how well prepared you are – how many questions you've written down, how carefully you've tracked your cycles, how respectful your tone – there may still come a moment when you feel it: that sudden shift in energy. The consultant glancing at the clock. The nurse brushing off your concerns. The administrator speaking to you like you're being difficult for simply asking about costs or timelines. In that moment, the room may feel colder. Your voice may feel smaller. And you might wonder: *Is it just me?*

It's not just you.

The fertility system is overburdened. But that does not excuse poor communication or emotional insensitivity. You are allowed to expect more than efficiency - you are allowed to expect *care*.

Feeling unheard or dismissed by your care team can shake your trust, especially when you've placed something as sacred and vulnerable as your family-building journey in their hands. The first step is to **recognise the signs**. Dismissal can be overt, but often, it's subtle:

- Repeatedly interrupting you or ignoring your questions
- Talking *about* you instead of *to* you
- Using overly technical jargon without checking your understanding
- Rolling eyes, sighing, or making you feel like a burden
- Failing to follow up on promised information

These behaviours may not be intentional, but their impact is real. And if left unaddressed, they can lead to miscommunication, emotional distress, and even poor outcomes.

When this happens, you have options. The first is to gently but clearly **name the issue**. This doesn't mean confrontation - it means clarity. Phrases like:

- "I want to make sure I'm understanding you correctly – could we slow down a little?"
- "I feel like my concerns weren't fully addressed just now. Could we revisit that point?"
- "I'm finding this conversation difficult. Would it be possible to schedule a follow-up so I can digest this information first?"

Sometimes, naming the dynamic shifts it immediately. Other times, it reveals a pattern – one that may not change, no matter how politely you ask. In those cases, it's important to **document** your experiences. Keep a log of what was said, when, and how it made you feel. This isn't about building a case, necessarily – it's about having a record that helps you make future decisions with confidence.

If a provider repeatedly dismisses your concerns, it is absolutely within your rights to request a different clinician. You don't need to justify this with a dramatic story. A simple statement like "I feel I would benefit from a fresh perspective" is enough. And if the clinic resists or refuses – that's a red flag. You deserve a team that respects your voice as part of your care plan.

One woman I supported was told by her consultant, after a failed round, "Some people just don't respond well, and that's the end of it." She left the clinic in tears, believing her only option was to give up. After encouragement, she sought a second opinion. The new clinic changed her protocol, listened carefully, and helped her feel like a partner – not a problem. It wasn't just about clinical expertise. It was about **respect**.

Of course, speaking up is not always easy - especially when emotions are high and power dynamics are at play. That's where having **scripts and support** helps. Practice what you want to say before appointments. Roleplay with a friend. Write down your points and bring them in. You don't have to be eloquent - you just have to be honest.

If you experience overt disrespect, discrimination, or negligence, you can also file a formal complaint. Every clinic should have a Patient Liaison or complaint process. It may not change what happened, but it creates a record. And it may lead to policy changes that help others. You are not being "difficult." You are upholding standards that should already exist.

Sometimes, the most powerful response to not being heard is to **move your care entirely**. Yes, it takes effort. Yes, it may cost more. But your peace of mind - your ability to trust your providers and feel safe in their hands - is worth protecting. You don't owe loyalty to a clinic that doesn't see you. You owe yourself kindness, clarity, and a team who treats you like a whole person, not just a patient number.

You might feel exhausted by this work. It's okay to feel that way. Self-advocacy is not a personality trait - it's a skill. And like all skills, it gets easier with practice. Every time you clarify your needs, every time you ask a question, every time you choose presence over passivity, you strengthen that muscle.

And perhaps most importantly: **you are not being dramatic. You are not overreacting. You are not too sensitive.**

You are someone fighting to become a parent - in a system that does not always make room for your voice.

As we close this chapter, we move from navigating clinical conversations to understanding your legal and financial rights as a fertility patient. In Chapter Eight, we'll look at what protections, policies, and patient rights exist – and how to use them to your advantage when the process feels stacked against you.

9

Know Your Rights: Understanding Your Protections, Policies, and Power

What You're Entitled To - The Legal Landscape of IVF

When you're standing at the threshold of something as intimate and life-altering as IVF, it's easy to forget that the journey isn't just emotional - it's also legal, logistical, and bound by a framework of rights and protections. The trouble is, these rights are rarely spelled out. They're tucked away in fine print, assumed knowledge, or buried in the terms and conditions you clicked "agree" to in a fog of hope.

But you *do* have rights. As a fertility patient, a healthcare consumer, and a person making deeply personal decisions about your future, you are protected by more than just trust. You're protected - or should be - by law, policy, and standards of care.

This section brings those rights into the light. Because when you understand them, you no longer have to ask permission to be treated with dignity. You can *expect it.*

Let's start with the basics: depending on where you live, **fertility services may be governed by national or regional health laws**. These laws define everything from clinic licensing and patient privacy to consent procedures, record keeping, and how embryos are stored or disposed of.

In the UK, for example, clinics must be licensed by the Human Fertilisation and Embryology Authority (HFEA), which sets out strict regulations on:

- Informed consent for every stage of treatment
- Storage limits for embryos and gametes
- Clinic success rate reporting
- Advertising standards
- Psychological support availability

In the US, there's no single federal oversight body, but individual states have varying regulations, and clinics must comply with HIPAA privacy laws and relevant consumer protections. Australia has the NHMRC ethical guidelines and state-level laws. Canada, too, is provincially governed, with Assisted Human Reproduction Canada setting national frameworks.

The specifics vary, but the principles should not: **you have the right to accurate information, clear consent procedures, protection of your medical data, and respectful care.**

What does that mean in practice?

First, it means you have the right to **clear, jargon-free explanations** of your treatment, including:

- Why a particular protocol is being recommended
- What the risks and benefits are
- What alternatives exist (including doing nothing)
- What it will cost - not just upfront, but in follow-up procedures, storage, medication, and exit fees

If this isn't offered freely, ask. If it still isn't forthcoming, you can and should escalate your request to clinic management or the appropriate regulatory body. You are not asking for a favour - you are requesting transparency, which is a *legal and ethical requirement.*

Second, you have the right to **control what happens to your reproductive material** - your eggs, sperm, and embryos. This includes:

- Deciding how long they're stored (within legal limits)
- Withdrawing consent at any time
- Specifying what happens to embryos in case of death, separation, or end of treatment

These are deeply emotional issues, and it can feel jarring to encounter legal documents around them. But knowing your rights here protects you later - especially in cases of disagreement or clinic mismanagement.

Third, you have the right to **access your medical records**, including test results, treatment notes, and lab reports. In many countries, this is not only a right but a legal guarantee. Clinics may charge a small administrative fee, but they cannot withhold this information. Having access to your full record allows you to seek second opinions, double-check your history, and make informed decisions about next steps.

It also means you have the right to **privacy and dignity** throughout treatment. That includes:

- Not being asked invasive or irrelevant questions
- Being addressed by your correct name and pronouns
- Having space for emotional processing
- Being offered support services if available

If you ever feel these rights are violated, you can file a complaint with the governing body for your clinic. This might be the HFEA, a state medical board, or a consumer protection office. You don't need to have suffered physical harm to make a complaint. Emotional distress, discriminatory treatment, or financial misrepresentation are all legitimate concerns.

This is especially important in cases involving **discrimination**. Fertility services are not just for one kind of person or family. Clinics cannot legally discriminate based on marital status, sexual orientation, gender identity, disability, or race. Yet we know that many do - subtly or overtly - through gatekeeping, pricing disparities, or unequal emotional support.

If you experience this, you are not overreacting. You are

encountering systemic bias that has no place in reproductive healthcare. And you are entitled to challenge it - publicly or privately - as you see fit.

One woman I spoke to was told, bluntly, that pursuing IVF as a single woman "wouldn't be worth it" for someone her age. She left the clinic shaken, but later discovered she had the legal right to access services without a partner, and found a clinic that welcomed her fully. What changed wasn't her eligibility - it was her *awareness*.

Of course, rights on paper don't always translate into reality. That's where **knowing who to contact** becomes vital. Keep a short list:

- Your country's fertility regulator (e.g. HFEA, ASRM, or equivalent)
- A patient advocacy group or ombudsman
- A legal advice service that specialises in reproductive health

You may never need to use them. But knowing they're there can bring a quiet kind of power - the kind that reminds you you're not just navigating treatment. You're participating in a system. And systems can be held accountable.

As we continue this chapter, we'll explore how insurance policies, payment plans, and employer benefits interact with your rights - and how to make sure the financial aspects of treatment are just as transparent and fair as the clinical ones.

Insurance, Costs, and What You Shouldn't Have to Fight For

There's a particular kind of exhaustion that sets in when you're doing everything right, and still can't get a straight answer. You've read the clinic's brochures. You've asked for a breakdown. You've called your insurance provider three times this week, spoken to five different people, and heard five different answers. And somehow, amidst all this, you're still expected to inject yourself on schedule, show up emotionally prepared, and keep your finances afloat. It's not just stressful – it's surreal.

The financial side of IVF is often the most opaque part of the entire process. Clinics advertise "package deals," but what exactly do they include? Insurance coverage is referenced vaguely, with disclaimers longer than any assurance. And worst of all, you may feel like you're being impolite – or pushy – simply for asking, *"Can you walk me through what this will actually cost?"*

But here's the truth: transparency is not a favour. It's a right. And while the healthcare industry may not always act like it, financial clarity should be part of informed consent – just as much as knowing your medical risks or treatment options.

Let's start with **insurance coverage**, since it's often the most confusing terrain. In the United States, only about 20 states have laws requiring some level of infertility insurance coverage, and even within those, the policies vary dramatically. Some states mandate only that diagnostic testing be covered. Others extend to treatment, but not medications. Some require proof of failed attempts before coverage kicks in. Some exclude same-sex couples or single parents altogether.

In countries like the UK, Australia, or Canada, national or

regional health services may cover parts of the fertility process, but there are often strict eligibility requirements - based on age, BMI, prior children, and more.

So your first step is to **get crystal clear** on your personal situation. This means requesting your insurance plan's Explanation of Benefits (EOB), ideally in writing, and sitting down with someone - a benefits advisor, a clinic finance specialist, or even a trusted friend - to go through it slowly. You are looking for specific answers to questions like:

- Are fertility *diagnostics* covered, even if treatment isn't?
- Is IVF, IUI, or egg freezing part of the policy - and are there limits?
- Are medications billed through pharmacy benefits or medical?
- Is prior authorisation required for any stage of care?
- What are the lifetime or cycle maximums?
- What documentation is required to qualify for coverage?

You may need to call your provider directly, and that's okay. Just remember: their job is to inform you. You do not need to apologise for asking twice - or five times - if the answers are unclear.

Now, let's turn to **clinic pricing**. Many fertility clinics operate as private practices, even within national health systems. That means they set their own fees and billing structures - and it's up to *you* to ask for clarity.

You have the right to request:

- A full, itemised price list
- A written quote for your proposed treatment plan
- A breakdown of what is included in any "package" or bundle
- The cost of medications, monitoring, storage, anaesthesia, and lab work – all separately listed
- Details of cancellation or rescheduling fees, including what happens if your cycle is delayed or cancelled due to poor response

If the clinic is hesitant to provide this, or gives you a vague "it depends," that is not acceptable. It is perfectly reasonable – and smart – to say, "Before I commit to this plan, I'd like a written outline of all possible charges."

Some clinics will present optional add-ons – such as assisted hatching, time-lapse embryo imaging, or endometrial scratching – with little evidence of efficacy. These extras can add thousands to your bill, yet offer marginal or no proven benefit. You are not being a bad patient if you decline them. You are being an informed one.

One couple I worked with was encouraged to add on every possible test "just in case," bringing their out-of-pocket quote from £5,000 to over £12,000 – without a clear explanation. They paused, took the time to research each add-on, and discovered that most weren't medically necessary for their case. When they returned to the clinic with questions, they were met with defensiveness. They changed clinics – and saved nearly £6,000 in the process.

That's not luck. That's clarity.

Now let's talk about **your own budgeting safeguards**. First, consider setting up a simple spreadsheet or notebook log where you track every cost related to your treatment:

- Clinic consultations and procedures
- Medication purchases
- Bloodwork, ultrasounds, and lab fees
- Embryo freezing and annual storage
- Travel or accommodation (if needed)
- Counselling or support services

It might feel overwhelming at first, but this log becomes your financial foundation. When a surprise invoice arrives, or when a billing error occurs, you have a record to refer to - and challenge if needed.

You also have the right to **compare pricing between clinics**, even if you've already begun consultations with one. Some regions offer significant savings by travelling for treatment - either to different states or even countries with strong medical reputations. Fertility tourism is not for everyone, and it carries additional logistical and emotional challenges, but it's a valid option, especially when cost is a major barrier.

If you're working, consider whether your employer offers **separate fertility benefits** through companies like Progyny, Maven, or Carrot. These platforms often cover specific services outside traditional insurance, including egg freezing, IVF cycles, donor sperm or eggs, and more. If your employer doesn't offer such benefits, it is increasingly acceptable - and effective - to advocate for them. Some companies have added fertility coverage in response to just a few employee requests.

Finally, let's talk about your **financial dignity**. You are allowed to say, "This is too much." You are allowed to pause. You are allowed to make choices based not just on hope, but on sustainability. Budgeting is not giving up - it's *staying in the game longer.*

Transparency is the foundation of trust. If a provider, clinic, or policy asks you to move forward without it - pause. Ask again. You are not a number. You are not a chart. You are a person planning a future family with care and intelligence. You deserve honesty - and answers.

In the final section of this chapter, we'll explore what happens when your rights are denied altogether - and what steps you can take to stand your ground, be heard, and keep your peace even when systems fall short.

When the System Fails - Escalation, Advocacy, and Protecting Your Peace

There's a moment that many people face on the IVF journey that no one warns you about. It's not the moment of loss, or waiting, or even heartbreak. It's the moment when you realise you've done everything right - followed every instruction, paid every invoice, showed up with your body and heart wide open - and still, something deeply unfair has happened. A bill you weren't told about. A decision made without your consent. A tone of voice from a provider that left you feeling small and silenced.

And you find yourself thinking, *Surely this can't be how it works?*

But too often, it is. The fertility industry is not always patient-first. And while many clinics offer ethical, compassionate care, the system as a whole is not built to protect you - unless you know how to stand your ground.

When things go wrong, most people's instinct is to try harder: to be nicer, to ask more politely, to send another follow-up. And sometimes, that works. But sometimes, the system fails in a way that no amount of grace can fix.

That's when you escalate.

Escalation doesn't mean being combative. It means choosing clarity over confusion, boundaries over burnout. It means understanding that being a "good" patient doesn't mean being a quiet one.

If something happens in your care that feels unsafe, inappropriate, financially misleading, or emotionally harmful, **you have the right to file a formal complaint**. Not as a last resort, but as a legitimate next step in seeking accountability.

Start by requesting your clinic's internal complaints procedure. Reputable providers should offer this freely - if they don't, that's a red flag in itself. Ask:

- Who handles patient complaints?
- What is the expected timeline for a response?
- Will your care be affected by submitting a complaint?

Then, document what happened:

- Dates, times, names of staff involved
- What was said, promised, or done
- What the impact was (emotionally, financially, medically)
- What resolution you're requesting (apology, refund, policy change, transfer of care)

Keep your language clear and factual, but don't leave out emotional truth. You are not being petty by describing how you were made to feel. Respectful complaints can - and should - include the human impact.

If the clinic's response is inadequate or dismissive, **you don't have to accept that as the end of the story**. Every country has oversight bodies for healthcare services:

- In the UK: the Human Fertilisation and Embryology Authority (HFEA)
- In Australia: State Health Complaints Entities or the Australian Health Practitioner Regulation Agency (AHPRA)
- In Canada: Provincial Colleges of Physicians and Surgeons
- In the US: State medical boards, the American Society for Reproductive Medicine (ASRM), or insurance regulators

These bodies exist to protect standards – and to hear your voice when others won't. You can also contact legal aid organisations that specialise in reproductive health if your case involves discrimination or breach of contract.

One patient, a single woman in her late 30s, was pressured to sign a storage agreement that would have automatically transferred embryo ownership to her clinic after two years if she couldn't pay renewal fees. She questioned it, and was told "That's just how we do things." But she researched her rights, contacted her country's health ombudsman, and found that the clause violated national reproductive law. She challenged the clinic. The clause was removed.

Her embryos – and her autonomy – were protected not by luck, but by knowledge.

Not every escalation will lead to immediate change. Sometimes the system drags its feet. Sometimes the most important shift is not in the clinic's policy, but in your own decision to move on.

Because you can do that, too. If trust has been broken beyond repair, **you have the right to transfer your care**. You can request your complete medical file, including:

- Hormone levels
- Procedure notes
- Embryo grading and storage reports
- Scan results
- Consent forms and financial statements

In many countries, clinics are legally obligated to provide this within a set timeframe. You don't need to justify your choice. You are simply protecting your wellbeing.

But perhaps the hardest system to push back against is the internal one – the voice that says, *Maybe I'm overreacting. Maybe I'm too sensitive. Maybe it's not that bad.*

Let me be clear: **you are not too sensitive** for wanting to be treated with respect. You are not difficult for expecting clear answers. You are not wrong to say, *No more surprises, no more shame, no more silence.*

Your peace matters.

And sometimes, the most powerful act of advocacy is not writing a complaint or quoting policy – it's choosing to rest. To heal. To say, *I need a break from being in fight mode.*

That may mean stepping away for a cycle. It may mean switching clinics. It may mean grieving the way you hoped to feel about this experience – and making space for the more complicated truth.

There is no shame in having to push back. There is no failure in feeling tired of pushing. There is only a quiet, fierce kind of strength in knowing that you are still here, still asking questions, still fighting – not just for a baby, but for yourself.

And that is enough.

In the next chapter, we'll step back from the systems and return to your own centre. We'll explore how to stay connected to your body, your identity, and your inner compass – even when the world around you makes that difficult.

10

Staying Connected: Reclaiming Your Body, Identity, and Power in the Process

The Emotional Cost of IVF - and How to Honour It

No one tells you how loud the silence can be.

The silence after an early morning scan when the clinic is too busy to offer more than a rushed, "We'll call you."

The silence in the car ride home, as you sit beside your partner, both too cautious to say what you're feeling.

The silence when you lie in bed wondering, *What if this doesn't work? What then?*

IVF is a medical process – but it doesn't feel like medicine. Not in the way we're taught to expect. There are no crisp diagnoses followed by clear cures. No promises, no guarantees. Just hope, held loosely. A series of small steps that may lead somewhere beautiful, or nowhere at all.

And throughout that journey, your body becomes a landscape of effort. Bruised injection sites. Bloating from hormones. Endless blood draws. Vaginal probes. The sharp inhale of the word "unfortunately" during a call you didn't want to answer.

These are not just physical tolls. They are emotional imprints. And too often, we're taught to overlook them - to treat them as "part of the process," to focus on the outcome, to be strong, brave, resilient. As though resilience means pretending nothing hurts.

But the emotional cost of IVF is real. It is not weakness. It is not drama. It is a legitimate part of the experience - one that deserves space, care, and compassion.

Grief is a quiet companion in this process. Not always dramatic, but ever-present. Grief for the time passing. Grief for the ease others seem to have. Grief for the version of yourself that once believed it might happen differently. Some days it shows up as fatigue. Some days as irritability. Some days as numbness so deep you wonder if you'll ever feel "normal" again.

This grief needs witnessing. And that witnessing must start with you.

One of the most powerful things you can do in IVF is not push through, but *pause within.* To give yourself the dignity of honesty - to say, *This is hard,* without immediately following it with, *but I'm fine.* To let your sorrow breathe.

That doesn't mean surrendering to despair. It means making room. Emotional processing is not a detour from the path - it's part of the way forward.

So what does it look like to honour the emotional cost of IVF?

It starts with validation. You don't need someone else's permission to feel what you feel. You don't need your experience to be the worst, the longest, the most dramatic, to deserve empathy. Pain is not a competition. It's a human response to unmet expectations, to loss, to longing, to uncertainty.

And you are allowed to grieve even in the midst of hope. Hope does not cancel out sorrow – they can sit side by side. You can hope fiercely and still weep when another cycle doesn't go to plan. You can celebrate one embryo and still ache for the ones that didn't make it. Complexity is not contradiction. It's honesty.

Journaling can be one of the gentlest tools for this kind of honesty. Not a neat, curated journal – but a raw, unfiltered space where no thought is too messy to record. Write without editing. Let the page catch what your mind can't hold alone.

Some days, writing may help. Other days, silence may feel safer. On those days, honour your body in other ways: a long bath, a walk with no destination, music that meets your mood instead of trying to change it.

You might also find comfort in small rituals – not to fix the pain, but to mark it. Lighting a candle for a cycle that's ended. Keeping a stone in your pocket to ground you during appointments. Planting something that grows slowly, like lavender or rosemary, as a living symbol of patience.

These gestures aren't performative. They're personal. They remind you that *you* are still here. That your worth isn't tied to results. That you are more than the process unfolding around you.

IVF can make you feel like a vessel – useful only if you deliver. But you are not a vessel. You are a whole person, living a whole life, even in this liminal space.

Connection begins with that remembering. And in the next section, we'll explore what it means to reconnect with your body – not as a failing machine, but as a partner in this process, worthy of tenderness, trust, and love.

Reconnecting with Your Body - Moving from Surveillance to Self-Compassion

There's a moment, somewhere in the middle of a fertility cycle, when your body no longer feels like yours. You've measured it, injected it, scanned it, reported on it. You've watched it swell, react, and disappoint. Your body becomes a project – monitored and managed, observed and assessed. Its worth reduced to follicle counts, lining thickness, hormone levels.

And slowly, subtly, your language shifts. You talk about it as if it's separate from you. *"My body isn't responding." "It's not doing what it should."* You begin to mistrust it. Or worse – to resent it.

That quiet separation can be one of the most painful parts of IVF. Because it's not just about biology. It's about identity. If your body is failing at the very thing it was "supposed" to do – what does that make you?

But here's what the clinics don't tell you, and what the glossy brochures don't show: your body is not failing. It is trying. It is enduring. It is showing up every single day under conditions no one would choose. It is surviving – and you are surviving with it.

Reconnecting with your body after – or during – fertility treatment is not easy. It is not linear. But it is possible. And more than that, it is healing. Because your body is not just a site of medical intervention. It is your home. It deserves love, even now.

The first step in that reconnection is shifting the narrative from **surveillance to support**.

Much of IVF trains us to observe the body like a technician. We're told to track, monitor, weigh, calculate. And in many ways, this is necessary – hormones and timing are crucial. But when observation becomes obsession, when every twinge is a sign, when every symptom is interpreted as success or failure – we lose ourselves.

So ask yourself: where can I step back from judgment, and step into kindness?

One woman shared with me that after months of daily symptom tracking, she took a break. She deleted the app. She stopped charting. She let herself feel what she felt, without assigning it a score. "I realised I didn't want my relationship with my body to feel like a report card anymore," she said. "I just wanted to be in it."

This is the shift: from data to dialogue. Instead of constantly measuring your body, speak to it. Thank it. Ask it what it needs.

You might be surprised by how much softer the process feels when you approach your body as a partner, not a puzzle.

Physical rituals can help rebuild this bond. Small, intentional acts that say, *I see you. I appreciate you. I'm still with you.* These might include:

- Gentle touch - placing your hands on your abdomen and breathing with intention
- Movement that feels expressive rather than corrective - dance, walking, stretching
- Rest that is guilt-free and restorative - naps, baths, doing nothing at all

You might also reclaim space through **clothing and environment**. During treatment, many people feel restricted - by waistbands, by medical gowns, by sterile rooms. At home, wear what feels comforting. Create corners of warmth - soft blankets, music you love, natural light, a scent that soothes you. These sensory details are small rebellions against the clinical.

Nutrition can also become a site of reconnection - not through strict regimes or moralised eating, but through nourishment. IVF can leave you feeling out of sync with your appetite, craving control where you can find it. Instead of following arbitrary rules, try asking your body what it truly wants. What would feel satisfying, energising, or grounding? This isn't about "fertility foods" - it's about dignity.

Of course, not all days will feel connected. There will be moments when your body feels like a stranger. When pain or bloating or exhaustion make kindness feel out of reach. That's okay. Reconnection isn't a destination – it's a practice. And like all practices, it allows for lapses.

If you're struggling, consider involving a professional – someone trained in body-based therapy, trauma-informed care, or somatic healing. These approaches can help you move gently back into your body, especially if medical experiences have made you feel dissociated or powerless.

And if therapy isn't accessible right now, turn to trusted companions. Sometimes, speaking aloud what you've only thought in private can shift the weight of it. A sentence like, "I'm angry at my body," can open a door – not to guilt, but to understanding.

One partner told me that what helped most wasn't fixing his wife's discomfort, but witnessing it. "She said, 'I feel like my body is betraying me.' I didn't argue. I didn't try to reassure her. I just said, 'I get that. I'm here with you.' That moment changed something."

You don't need perfect self-love. You just need presence. A willingness to stay with yourself, even when it hurts. Especially when it hurts.

Because here's the quiet truth: your body hasn't given up on you. It may be tired. It may be wounded. But it's still here. Still showing up. Still offering you breath, movement, heartbeat, life.

Let that be enough.

In the next and final section of this chapter, we'll explore how to reconnect with your identity outside of fertility - to rediscover who you are when you're not waiting, not hoping, not measuring. Just being.

Remembering Who You Are Beyond the Process

There's a particular kind of erosion that takes place during fertility treatment - not the sudden collapse of identity, but the slow, subtle wearing away of all the parts of yourself that once felt solid.

It starts with appointments. Schedules. Hormones. Blood tests. Before long, everything else - your hobbies, your creativity, your friendships, even your laughter - starts to fade into the background. Life gets quiet. Tighter. You shrink, not physically, but spiritually. Not because you've changed, but because everything else now seems to revolve around one question: *Will it work this time?*

And in that question, something else gets lost: *you.*

One of the most profound challenges of IVF is not just surviving the process - it's remembering that you exist *outside* of it. That there is more to you than the labels, the procedures, the calendar of medications. That before this began, you were already whole.

You had joy. Desire. Curiosity. A voice that spoke about more than follicles or fertility forums. You had a rhythm, a language, a taste for life that wasn't measured in hormone levels or clinic phone calls.

That version of you still exists. She's not gone – just quiet. And this chapter is an invitation to call her back.

Reconnecting with your identity is not about denying what you're going through. It's about expanding the lens. Saying: *Yes, this matters deeply – and so do I. All of me. Not just the part that's trying to conceive.*

One woman described it beautifully: "I realised I hadn't sung in months. Not in the car, not in the kitchen. I used to sing every day. And when I finally did, it was like a part of me reappeared – the part that wasn't waiting, wasn't calculating, just *being*."

Sometimes identity returns in quiet waves like that. Through a scent. A song. A familiar movement. A conversation that has nothing to do with fertility. Sometimes it comes through anger – the refusal to be reduced to a diagnosis. Sometimes it comes through softness – the gentle act of asking, *What do I want today that has nothing to do with this process?*

This kind of self-remembering can feel like rebellion – especially in a culture that equates womanhood with motherhood, worth with productivity, love with sacrifice. But it's not rebellion. It's repair.

You were never meant to be a vessel for someone else's timeline. You are not a blueprint waiting to be filled. You are a full story, already in progress.

So how do you begin to reconnect with that story?

First, reclaim your time. Even a few minutes a day that aren't tied to treatment can be sacred. Walk somewhere without your phone. Watch a film that makes you laugh – or sob. Write down three things about yourself that have nothing to do with your body. Remember the things that once lit you up, even if you don't feel ready to do them yet.

Next, allow your relationships to expand. During treatment, conversations can become narrowly focused. Every check-in becomes an update. "How's the cycle?" becomes the main thread. It's okay to say, "Can we talk about something else today?" It's okay to remind your friends and partner that you're still interested in their lives - and still want to share yours, too.

Identity also lives in your language. How do you talk about yourself? Is everything framed as "still trying," "waiting," "hoping"? See if you can introduce other words. "I'm also painting again." "I've started journaling." "I'm tired, but I'm proud of how I've coped." These small shifts are powerful. They signal to the world - and to your own mind - that you are not defined by this chapter alone.

Sometimes identity is recovered through boundaries. Choosing not to attend another baby shower. Unfollowing accounts that spark comparison. Declining conversations that leave you drained. These are not acts of bitterness. They are acts of protection.

One woman described her turning point like this: "I stopped explaining myself. I stopped making excuses for my choices. I just said, 'This is where I am right now.' And I felt so much lighter."

Reclaiming yourself also means allowing joy to return - even when it feels complicated. IVF often comes with a quiet guilt: how can I enjoy anything when I'm still waiting for *this*? But joy is not betrayal. Joy is resistance. It says: *I will not let this process take everything.*

So cook a meal that has nothing to do with "fertility nutrition." Book a weekend away if you can. Buy the dress. Make the art. Laugh loudly. Let yourself be messy and human and alive.

You do not owe the universe your suffering. You do not have to prove how much you want this by how much you sacrifice.

And if today all you can do is sit still and breathe - that counts, too.

You are not a before-and-after story. You are not a case study. You are a person in the middle of something immense. And the fact that you are still showing up - still asking questions, still making room for tenderness - is extraordinary.

In the next chapter, we'll explore what it means to open your heart to possibility - not just of pregnancy, but of family in all its forms. A hopeful, honest look at choice, chance, and the many paths to parenthood.

11

Embracing the Path Ahead: Redefining Hope, Family, and Enough

When the Picture Changes - Letting Go Without Giving Up

There's a photograph in your mind. A version of the future. It might be blurry around the edges or painstakingly detailed. A child's name. A house full of noise. A certain look exchanged across the dinner table on a sleepy Sunday morning. Whatever its form, it's more than just a wish - it's been a lighthouse guiding every decision, every injection, every appointment.

But sometimes, that picture changes.

Not because you gave up. Not because you didn't try hard enough. But because life has a way of taking the long road - the winding, unexpected, heartbreaking and heart-making route that few would choose but many must walk.

In this section, we begin with what is perhaps the most tender question of all: *What happens when the path shifts beneath you?*

It might begin subtly – a missed cycle, a delayed response to treatment, a conversation with your doctor that doesn't end with a plan but with a pause. Or it might come suddenly – a medical report that closes one door entirely. Either way, you're left standing in the rubble of a roadmap that no longer leads where you thought it would.

And the grief is sharp.

Not only because a dream is deferred, but because so much of your identity has been wrapped around it. Who are you if this version of the story doesn't unfold?

This is the moment when letting go begins.

But let's be clear – letting go is not the same as giving up. Letting go means creating room. Not to erase your desire, but to soften your grip on how it must arrive. Letting go is an act of courage, not defeat. It says: *I am still here, even as the picture shifts.*

One woman told me, "I thought if I let myself consider a different ending, it would mean I'd failed. But what I realised was, holding onto one version too tightly was breaking my heart more than the idea of change ever could."

Her path, eventually, led to donor conception. For someone else, it led to adoption. For another, it meant a conscious decision to live childfree – not because she didn't want children, but because she wanted herself more. Her health. Her partnership. Her peace.

There is no right answer. No moral hierarchy of family-making. Only what fits your life, your values, your needs – now, not five years ago. Letting go of one picture doesn't mean your story ends. It means you allow new images to emerge - ones you might never have imagined, but that are no less full of love.

To begin this shift, start by asking: *What am I holding onto out of fear, not truth?*

Are you afraid of what people will think? Of being judged, pitied, or questioned? Are you clinging to a particular route because it feels safer than facing the unknown?

It's okay if you are. You're human. But these questions can help loosen the grip - just enough to let air in.

Then ask: *What might be possible if I gave myself permission to want something different?*

Not because you're settling. But because you're evolving.

Sometimes it helps to write a letter - not to a baby or a clinic, but to yourself. The version of you who began this journey. Thank her. Mourn with her. Tell her what you know now. Let the writing be a bridge between then and now, between what was hoped for and what is becoming.

You might also choose to ritualise this shift. A small goodbye to the version of the story that's changing. One couple held a bonfire and burned the paperwork from their final failed cycle, then spent the evening telling stories of the life they still planned to build. Another woman planted a tree - not in memory of loss, but as a living symbol of what she was still growing: courage, clarity, resilience.

Letting go hurts. There is no way around that. But it also clears space. For rest. For reimagining. For new definitions of family, success, and enough.

In the next section, we'll gently explore what some of those definitions might be - including paths like donor conception, surrogacy, and adoption. Not as consolation prizes, but as real, rich, love-filled possibilities that might deserve a place in your story.

Expanding the Map - Donor Conception, Surrogacy, and Adoption

The path to parenthood, as the world often tells it, is narrow and straight: fall in love, get pregnant, raise a child. It's a story told in nursery rhymes and Instagram birth announcements. But the truth - the real truth - is much wider than that. It winds and forks and doubles back. Sometimes it crosses oceans. Sometimes it takes years. And sometimes, it opens into a new direction entirely.

For many people, reaching this place feels like both an ending and a beginning. The original plan has shifted. But that doesn't mean parenthood is no longer possible - only that its shape may change.

Let's begin with donor conception.

For some, this path becomes necessary when one partner's eggs or sperm are no longer viable - or when conception must happen without a partner at all. At first, the idea of involving a donor can feel clinical or complicated. But with time, many people come to see it for what it often becomes: an act of collaboration, of generosity, of creating life with the help of others.

There are choices to make. Will you use a known or anonymous donor? What kind of donor bank do you feel comfortable with? How will you talk to your future child about their origins?

These questions are real, and they deserve thoughtful answers. But they are not unsolvable. In fact, many families formed through donor conception are among the most intentional - parents who have faced every fork in the road, questioned every detail, and walked forward anyway.

One woman told me, "It used to break my heart that our baby wouldn't share my genetics. But now I realise they'll share my love, my laugh, my life. And that's what matters to me."

Then there's surrogacy - another path that is often misunderstood but deeply rooted in care. Surrogacy can take two forms: traditional (where the surrogate's own egg is used) or gestational (where the embryo is created using the intended parent's egg or donor egg). It can be altruistic, where the surrogate volunteers without compensation beyond expenses, or commercial, depending on the legal frameworks in your country.

Surrogacy requires trust. Communication. Legal clarity. Emotional honesty. It is not for everyone, and it involves complexities - financial, ethical, and logistical. But for some families, it is the door that finally opens after so many have closed.

It is also, fundamentally, a relationship. Between surrogate and intended parent. Between hope and reality. And when done ethically and transparently, it can be a profoundly healing experience for everyone involved.

One couple who pursued surrogacy after five failed IVF cycles described it like this: "Our surrogate didn't just carry our baby. She carried us. She gave us a way to believe again."

And then there is adoption.

Adoption is not the fallback option it's often portrayed to be – nor is it a shortcut to "having a baby." It is its own journey, with its own emotional terrain. It begins not with fertility, but with loss – the loss experienced by the child, the birth family, and often the adoptive parent as well.

But from that place, something new can grow. Something anchored in commitment, healing, and love.

If you're considering adoption, it's important to understand the different routes: domestic or international, infant or older child, open or closed adoption. Each comes with its own legal process, timeframes, and emotional landscapes. And each asks of you a specific kind of readiness – not just to parent, but to honour a child's history that didn't begin with you.

It's also worth saying: adoption is not a "cheaper" or easier version of parenting. It is a complex, lifelong commitment. But for those who feel called to it, it can be a homecoming – for both parent and child.

There's no hierarchy among these options. No gold star for one over another. Each carries its own beauty, challenge, and truth. The most important question is not *which is best* – but *which feels right for us, right now*?

And if none of these paths feel possible, or feel right – that, too, deserves respect. There is no failure in reaching the end of this road and saying, *This is where I stop.* You do not owe anyone a baby. You owe yourself honesty.

Every path has weight. Every decision has meaning. And every family - whether built through biology, generosity, partnership, or quiet choosing - is real.

In the final section of this chapter, we'll explore what it means to arrive at "enough." To stop chasing certainty, and instead make peace with the present - wherever it finds you.

Defining "Enough" - Peace, Closure, and the Life You're Living Now

There's a moment - and sometimes, it's so quiet you almost miss it - when you stop planning the next step. Not because you've lost hope. But because, for the first time in a long time, you feel a flicker of peace in simply being where you are.

It might come while sipping tea in the soft early light, when no one needs anything from you. Or in the middle of a conversation that's not about IVF at all. Or in the hush after a deep, cleansing cry. That moment, that pause, is where the idea of *enough* begins to take root.

In a world obsessed with optimization and achievement, "enough" can feel like a compromise. But in truth, it's a declaration of dignity. A gentle reclaiming of your boundaries, your body, your story. Not settling - but choosing. Not shrinking - but softening.

This section isn't about wrapping everything up with a neat bow. Fertility journeys rarely end cleanly. They leave traces – echoes of hope, sorrow, and everything in between. But even within that messiness, you can find meaning. You can arrive somewhere that feels livable. Spacious. Real.

So what does *enough* look like?

For some, it's a conscious decision to stop treatment – not because the desire for a child has faded, but because the toll has become too steep. Financially, emotionally, physically. They lay down the tools of the fight and pick up something quieter – rest, recovery, the rebuilding of a life not ruled by calendars and scans.

One woman shared, "I didn't stop because I no longer cared. I stopped because I wanted to care for myself again."

For others, *enough* comes in the form of family – but not the one originally imagined. A life with one child instead of two. A home filled with chosen family, pets, community. A new definition of legacy that has nothing to do with genetics, but everything to do with love.

Sometimes, *enough* is not a place you reach, but a feeling you begin to trust. A softening in your chest. A moment when you catch yourself smiling without explanation. A decision to redecorate the room you were saving as a nursery – not because you've given up, but because it deserves to be used now, not mourned forever.

This is not about erasing grief. There will still be pangs – birthdays not celebrated, holidays approached with a twinge of ache. But grief can live alongside joy. They are not mutually exclusive. The presence of longing does not cancel out the beauty of what you *do* have.

You might still light a candle for the embryos that never made it. Still flinch a little when another pregnancy announcement lands in your inbox. That's not failure. That's humanity.

In fact, making peace with "enough" requires radical compassion. It asks you to stop measuring your worth against outcomes. To stop waiting for permission to live fully. To stop tying your happiness to a future event.

It asks you to say: *This is my life. I will not wait to live it.*

And maybe - just maybe - it invites you to turn your attention outward. Toward others still in the trenches. Toward advocacy, support, or simply being the person who says, "I've been there." You don't owe your experience to anyone - but if and when you're ready, it can become a source of solidarity.

One couple I spoke with now hosts small gatherings for others navigating fertility decisions. They don't offer advice, just space. Tea, tissues, and time. "We wanted to create the room we never had," they said.

Your story may ripple in ways you'll never fully know. And your healing - quiet, unglamorous, and hard-won - is part of that ripple.

So, if no one has told you yet: you are allowed to rest. You are allowed to change your mind. You are allowed to feel joy. You are allowed to stop. You are allowed to carry on. You are allowed to hold conflicting emotions and still be whole.

You are allowed to define your own ending.

Or, perhaps, to realise there doesn't have to be one. Life will keep unfolding. Not as a straight line, but as a series of new beginnings.

This book may be closing. But your story is not over. It is expanding.

And wherever you go next – whether you continue to try, choose a new path, or decide to simply *be* – you are already enough.

12

The Journey You've Taken, and the One Still to Come

There's a quiet moment, after the research is done and the numbers have been run, after the questions and the doubts and the days of holding your breath – when all that remains is you. You, in your full, fierce, messy humanity. You, with your tender heart and your tired body. You, still standing.

This book wasn't meant to hand you answers in neat packages. Because there are none. Instead, it offered a way through – a path lined with truth, strategy, and care. A recognition that your longing is real, that your financial fears are valid, and that your hope deserves to be handled gently, not exploited.

You've moved through ten chapters of complexity. You've met your numbers with clarity. You've wrestled with systems and spreadsheets. You've imagined timelines and contingencies. You've fought for agency in rooms where you may have felt small. And all the while, you've carried something that doesn't show up on any receipt – your desire to build a family.

You've also learned how to hold your heart together when things fall apart. How to choose rest, even when everything tells you to keep pushing. How to speak up. How to let go – just a little – of shame. How to honour your body and remember who you are beyond this process.

That is no small thing.

If you're still in the thick of it – still calculating, still hoping – take this with you: it is okay to want what you want, and it is okay to want peace more.

If you've arrived at a different outcome than the one you imagined, let this book be a mirror that reflects your strength back to you. You made it through some of the hardest days with grace, even when it didn't feel graceful.

If you're somewhere in between – unsure, exhausted, undecided – may these pages remind you that you're not behind. You're becoming.

And wherever you are, may you know this:

You are not a statistic.

You are not a case file.

You are not a dollar amount on a clinic's ledger.

You are a person navigating one of life's most personal, and often most invisible, storms.

And you are doing it with astonishing courage.

Whether you become a parent in the way you originally dreamed, in a way you never expected, or not at all - your life still matters. Your story still matters. And your value was never tied to your reproductive outcome.

So, what now?

Maybe you pause. Maybe you talk to your partner. Maybe you look into funding options with fresh eyes. Maybe you reach out to someone who's been there. Maybe you close this book, exhale, and go for a walk. There's no single right next step - only the one that honours where you are right now.

This book has given you tools. But more than that, I hope it has given you permission. To hope. To grieve. To pivot. To rest. To redefine. To begin again.

The path ahead may not be clear - but you are not walking it empty-handed.

You carry knowledge. You carry perspective. You carry, above all, the right to shape your life with care.

And that is powerful.

Whatever tomorrow brings - know that you are not alone.

And know that you are enough.

13

A Note from the Author

Thank You, and What Comes Next

To whoever you are - the woman reading this quietly on her lunch break, the couple scrolling between appointments, the solo parent-to-be holding this book close like a conversation with someone who *gets it* - thank you.

Thank you for trusting me with your story, even for just a little while. I don't take it lightly. The journey you are on is deeply personal, often invisible to others, and frequently misunderstood. And yet, here you are - showing up. Seeking clarity. Choosing to meet this complex chapter with courage and care.

Writing this book was never about finding perfect solutions. It was about meeting real needs - financial, emotional, relational - with honesty, empathy, and actionable support. Because navigating IVF is not just about test results or protocols. It's about living inside uncertainty while still making plans. It's about holding on to hope without losing yourself.

If this book helped you feel less alone, more informed, or even just a little more grounded - then it has done its job.

As you close this book, I invite you to do three simple things:

- **Pause and honour how far you've come.**
- Even if the journey ahead feels long. Even if things are still undecided. You have done hard, brave things just by reading this far.

- **Share what helped you.**
- Whether it's a quote, a chapter, a budgeting idea, or a newfound perspective - someone else might need the same light you just found.

- **Stay connected to yourself.**
- Your body. Your voice. Your values. You are not just a vessel for someone else's timeline. You are a whole person, deserving of peace, support, and agency - now, not someday.

And when the noise gets loud, when the decisions pile up again, come back to this page if you need to. Let it remind you that you are doing better than you think.

A Handful of Affirmations to Take With You

You may want to copy them into your journal. Tape them to your mirror. Whisper them when the waiting gets heavy.

- I am allowed to want this, and I am allowed to take care of myself in the process.
- My worth is not measured in outcomes.
- I am doing the best I can with what I have.
- Rest is not weakness. It is wisdom.
- My body is not broken. It is doing its best under extraordinary pressure.
- I don't have to explain my path to anyone.
- I get to change my mind. I get to say no. I get to say, "this is enough."
- I am not alone.
- I am still becoming.

Thank you again for reading – and for being exactly who you are.
With all my warmth and admiration,

Alison
x

Printed in Dunstable, United Kingdom